CANNABIS SAVED MY LIFE

STORIES OF HOPE & HEALING

BY ELIZABETH LIMBACH

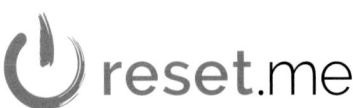

ISBN: 079484370-0
Printed in the United States of America
© 2016 reset.me

CONTENTS

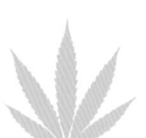

THE HUMAN EXPERIENCE OF MEDICINAL CANNABIS

It all started with one email.

It was a general query, addressed to a selection of acquaintances and organizations, explaining the premise of this book—that I was seeking Americans to talk about how cannabis impacted their health. I wrote the missive from the chatter-filled lair of a coffee shop in Santa Cruz, California, where I live, and hit send. (Not realizing until several of the email's recipients ribbed me about it later that it was sent at precisely *4:20* p.m.) As that initial invitation for prospective interviewees crossed the ethers, I wondered who I would profile in these pages. I worried that anyone I found wouldn't want his or her story immortalized in print. It is a sensitive subject, after all, one sometimes mired in legal complications.

I signed off and kept fretting—until I logged back on the following day and discovered an inbox brimming with replies. Brave people with ALS and MS and severe epilepsy and cancer and all manner of agonizing conditions wanted to share their story. They wanted to be heard.

Clearly, this was a subject close to many people's hearts. For those whose lives have been saved by this plant, telling their story is a way to help others open their hearts and minds to its potential, too.

It's also a chance for them to shed light on the obstacles and hypocrisies they have come up against along the way. Most of those featured on these pages tried cannabis only after exhausting all other options—after struggling through dozens of tried and failed treatments, surgeries and heavy-hitting pharmaceuticals. They overcame their own hesitations, social stigmas, the perils of illegality, and the disapproval of Western medicine to medicate with cannabis, and were met with astounding results. Having finally found the relief they sought, those living in states without medical marijuana laws became de facto criminals (and some were treated as such: read on to hear about devastatingly sick patients having their homes raided and medicine confiscated, then becoming enmeshed in legal woes), forcing many people to uproot or leave their families in order to relocate to a legal state. In conversations that were both haunting and inspirational, I found each person's story to be a testament to the strength of the human spirit in the bleakest of hours.

Viewed collectively, the profiles present a portrait not only of cannabis' promising abilities, but also of the problematically complex nature of our healthcare system and the pharmaceutical industry's chokehold on it. It also provides a peek at the dire consequences of marijuana prohibition. One mother's comment about this has been ringing in my ears ever since our interview, months ago: Heather Jackson's son, Zaki, spent much of his young life on the precipice of death, until cannabis finally controlled his seizures and gave him new life. "This isn't a political issue," Heather said. "This is a human rights issue. I want us to stop making political

decisions that could literally be life or death for a family."

What follows is decidedly anecdotal—frankly personal—looks at the human experience of medicinal cannabis, something that is often missing from broader conversations about the topic. It's an important ingredient for an educated discussion, as is research, which is mounting but badly needed in greater quantities (and this starts with the crucial precursor of funding for said research).

This brings to mind something another of the book's subjects, a formerly anti-marijuana mother with a host of painful disorders named Amy Echols, told me: "If I could go out and talk to anybody on the street, my advice would be to take your preconceived notions about cannabis, throw them out the window, and talk to people who are actual medical users." Here, I hope, is that chance.

— Elizabeth Limbach

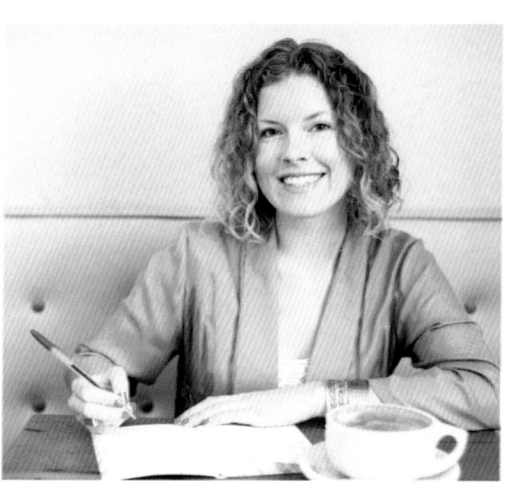

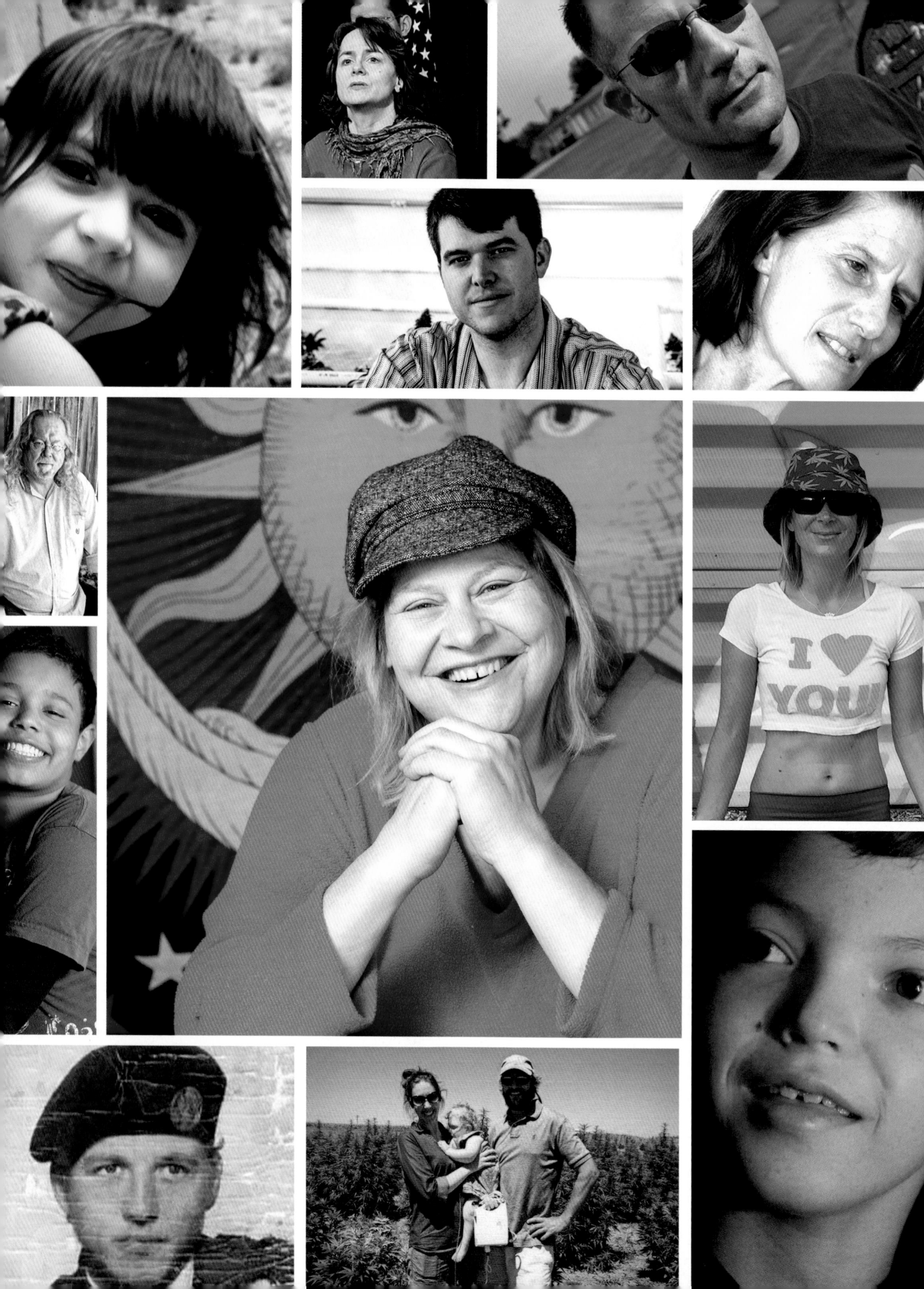

PROFILES
STORIES OF COURAGE

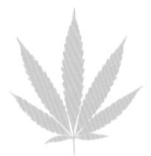

A.D.*

Age 47 / **PTSD, Head Injury** / Memphis, Tennessee

Soon after joining the Army at the age of 18, in 1987, A.D. realized it wasn't for him.

"I became more than disillusioned," says A.D. "It's hard to reconcile that. At some point, you have to figure out why you're even playing the game in order to fight, and sometimes it's hard to come up with that reason."

A.D., who served in the Army until 1991, during which time he was stationed at Fort Bragg in Northern California, believes that the aggressive, violence-condoning military culture is at the root of his PTSD, not necessarily the specific settings and experiences he had while serving.

"No matter whether you went to combat or not, when you're in the military, violence is contagious and addictive, and not everybody gets over not being able to do that stuff anymore [once they are out]," he says. "I've seen firsthand just how

crazy things get when you're around people who are addicted to violence."

Surviving the military experience meant keeping quiet about this type of behavior and about any injuries he incurred that weren't visibly drastic. It also meant taking any number of prescription drugs doled out to him.

In 1988, A.D. caught a roundhouse kick on the side of the head while playing soccer. He tried to shake it off. "Our culture is such that if you get hurt, you pretty much have to be holding one of your arms that's fallen off in the other arm for anyone to understand you're hurt," he says. He suffered a traumatic brain injury as a result of that kick, which changed his field of vision. When he left the Army, he was given a disability level of 10 percent because of his vision problems, but the head injury was never addressed.

"I've received so many diagnoses from so many different doctors at the VA

*A.D. LIVES IN A STATE WHERE MOST FORMS OF CANNABIS USE ARE ILLEGAL, AND HE HAS REQUESTED TO BE IDENTIFIED BY HIS INITIALS FOR SAFETY REASONS.

"I HAVE TO MOVE HALFWAY ACROSS THE COUNTRY SO I DON'T HAVE TO WORRY ABOUT BEING A CRIMINAL."

that, for the longest time, I didn't know what was wrong with me," he says, citing depression and narcolepsy as some of the things he was treated for. "Throughout my 30s, the medications they were giving me were driving me crazy."

He was prescribed amphetamines to stay awake during the day and Klonopin to sleep at night, as well as anti-psychotics, Ritalin, and more. "They were trying to turn me into a crackhead," he says. In the darkest hour, he was unable to find a job and struggled with homelessness.

As he neared 40 years old, A.D. discovered cannabis' medical applications while on the hunt for something to stimulate his appetite, which was feeble. He says that cannabis has allowed him to treat his issues without damaging his organs like the VA-endorsed medicines did, and has made it possible to live a full life without the hampering anxiety and tension he inherited from his time in the Army. Over the course of several years using cannabis, he weaned himself from the 12 different prescribed medications he was taking daily.

"It [cannabis] has given me the ability to have honest emotions, to be present with the people I'm with," he says. "I can pay attention to people long enough to listen to their jokes without hearing a

twig snap in the woods 30 feet behind them and wonder what it is. My kidneys don't hurt anymore, I'm no longer constantly constipated—there's a whole lot of stuff that doesn't happen anymore."

Medicating is risky for A.D., however, because he lives in Tennessee, which currently only allows for its use in high-CBD form for intractable seizures. He is weighing the pros and cons of relocating to Colorado, where medical marijuana is legal, and says it's starting to feel like he doesn't have a choice: in Tennessee, he has to make illicit drug deals to obtain his medicine. In Colorado, he could safely and legally buy medicine.

"I have to move halfway across the country so I don't have to worry about being a criminal," he says. "I'd like to live here, where I have the love and support of my family and friends."

He hopes that someday veterans can receive treatment like he has with cannabis that will allow them to heal, not make their struggles worse. "We're the people you see every day," he says. "The guy who delivers your water. The guy dropping off your package. It's not just the guys dressed in camouflage, sleeping on the streets. That's the end result of what happens after years of taking those [prescription] drugs—*after* you go through all of that."

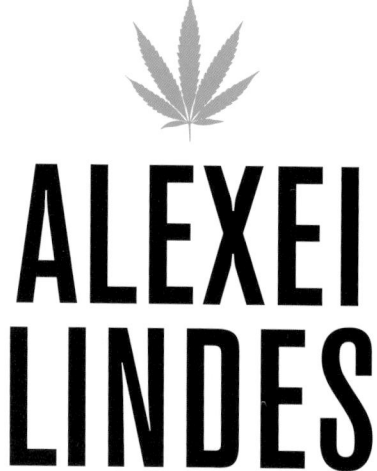

ALEXEI LINDES

Age 33 / **Complex PTSD** / Reno, Nevada

By the time Alexei Lindes entered his teen years, his parents and teachers didn't know what to do with him.

He pulled the fire alarm at school and yelled at the principal. He was expelled on several occasions, and ran away from home more than a dozen times. He was out of control, and no one in his life seemed to know how to help—or, perhaps, cared to really figure it out.

"I was quite defiant and not able to fit into the normal status quo," says Alexei, who is now a 33-year-old massage therapist in Reno, Nevada.

Several times, his parents responded to his problems by placing him in the UCLA psychiatric unit. It was during one of these hospitalizations, on a summer night in 1996, that two unfamiliar men entered the 14-year-old's room and told him to get dressed.

His questions went unanswered and he was ordered to "be quiet" as he pulled on his clothes, then was escorted to a waiting SUV, which wound through the dark city to LAX airport.

Still unsure of what was happening or why, he was soon at a residential treatment center for teens in Provo, Utah, where he lived until three days before his 18th birthday.

"My life before that ceased to exist the second I went there," says Alexei. He spent the next four years in a pharmaceutical haze, slogging between his four-person dorm room, class, and the many activities and chores meant to help treat him. He saw his parents, who had

"I REMEMBER GOING OUT TO A COFFEE SHOP FOR THE FIRST TIME AND SITTING WITH A FRIEND. I WAS HAVING COFFEE AND SITTING OUTSIDE AND I WAS NOT TERRIFIED OF SOMETHING ATTACKING ME."

sent him to the facility, just a handful of times during his stay.

The center ran on a system of earning and losing privileges. This was dictated by a point scale, which had the children on a constant seesaw between five levels, each with its own set of rules meant to reflect the shame or pride of having dipped or ascended to that particular level. At Level One, Alexei explains, he wasn't allowed to speak. One bracket up, he could talk, but was not permitted to go outdoors. When gracing the top of the behavioral hierarchy, at Level Five, he was expected to restrain and discipline other kids. These standings were delicate—changes were swift and volatile.

"This would cause a lot of frustration because you could be working hard and being really good for months on end and get up to Five, and then one little thing would take you down to a One," Alexei says. Being distracted in class or a misstep during a chore brought punishment, including "a day, or weeks, or months" in isolation. "I knew kids who practically lived down there," he says.

The decisions were issued in a seemingly desultory manner that Alexei says kept him in a state of constant anxiety and fear. As the years went on, he saw them as part of a broader strategy to keep residents raw and afraid.

"I witnessed a lot of physical abuse on a daily basis, but it was mostly emotional—the breaking down and supposedly building up of your character," he says. "Anything goes at these places."

The psychological damage of this compounded over time, exacerbated by scarring stints in isolation and the gradual trauma of living each day in fear, waiting for the situation to "go awry" again, as he knew it could at any moment.

A cumulative unease took root deep within Alexei. But upon moving back to his parents' home in the year 2000, at the age of 18, the insidious sprouts of this discomfort had yet to pierce the surface. In fact, for the first few months of his homecoming, it appeared as if the program had really worked.

"It seemed like I'd been built up to be perfect, and everything *was* perfect," he says. "And then it all fell apart like a house of cards."

Alexei was alienated and frustrated. He didn't have anyone to talk to about what he'd been through, and couldn't have if he wanted to—he didn't yet have the language or tools to understand it himself. The unsettling feelings erupted

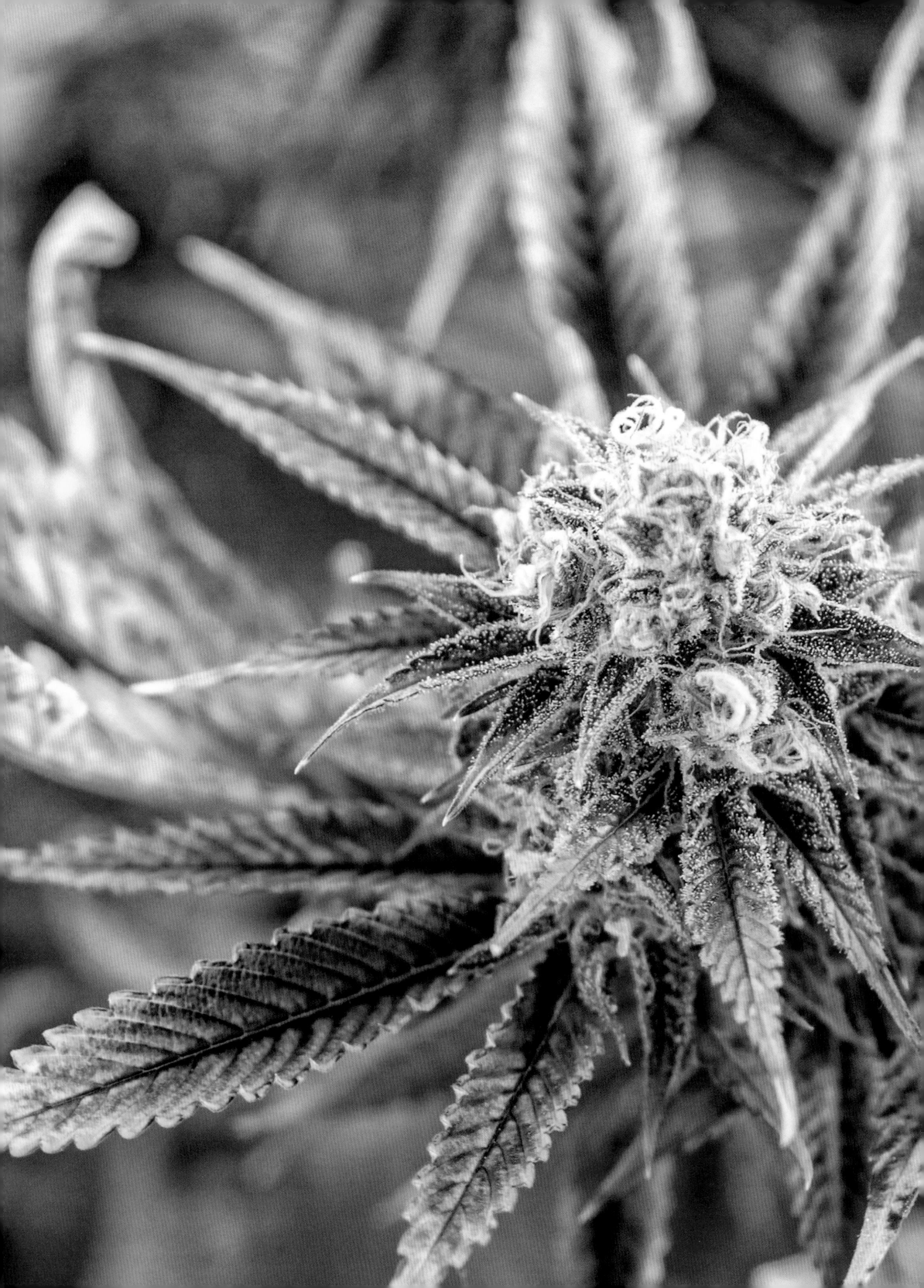

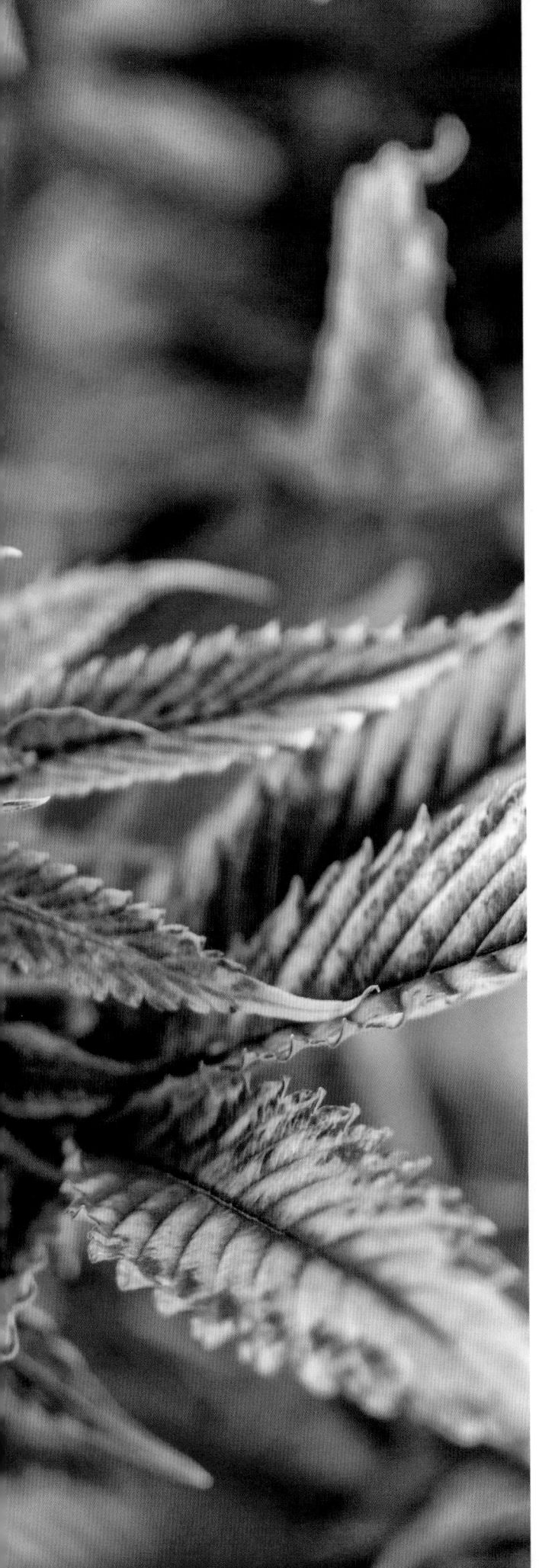

AT HIS PEAK, ALEXEI LINDES SUFFERED UP TO 20 PANIC ATTACKS EVERY DAY. UPON TRYING MEDICAL MARIJUANA, THE ATTACKS BECAME LESS FREQUENT—DROPPING TO ONE A MONTH, AND THEN ONE EVERY SIX MONTHS, UNTIL THEY CEASED ALTOGETHER. IT HAS BEEN THREE YEARS SINCE HIS LAST ATTACK.

from within as anxiety, depression and stress. He began to have panic attacks—one or two a day at first, and then 10, or 15, or 20. For anywhere from five to 30 minutes, he suffocated under what felt like "a 300-pound person sitting on my chest."

"It was all of the racing thoughts of panic and not being able to figure out how to cope with whatever physically was going on," he says. "It felt like I was drowning." He would pop a Klonopin or another benzodiazepine prescribed to him for such situations, adding to his ongoing high-dose regime of Zoloft and Seroquel.

"I REMEMBER BEING ELATED AND HAVING A FEELING OF RELIEF."

His requests to his psychiatrist for lower dosages were refused, leaving him with the option of facing a full day of attacks unmedicated or "drooling at the wall." Terrified of suffering through an episode in public, Alexei would not go outside for weeks at a time.

"I was not living a normal life at all," he says.

Cannabis wasn't a possibility for Alexei, whose strict residential treatment experience had scared him out of ever trying it.

"I'd had this thing pummeled into my head for four years that if I did pot I'd become a drug addict and homeless and out of control, so I was extremely fearful of pot," he explains. "Previous offers had come by that I'd declined."

Perhaps it was fate, then, that he happened to ingest it for the first time by accident. One evening, a guest brought marijuana brownies to a party that his mother hosted. Unwitting, Alexei ate one. A social setting like a party would usually trigger a panic attack for Alexei, who would retreat to his room to deal with it in private. On this night, however, the inevitable attack never materialized. Against all odds, he found himself socializing—and *enjoying* it.

"I remember being elated and having a feeling of relief," he says. "It was beauti-ful. It was like nothing else." A few hours later, he told his mother how he was feeling and she deduced what had happened.

"I had a moment of 'Oh my God, I just took marijuana and I'm going to be an addict now,'" he remembers. "Then I realized that was silly because I wasn't behaving like a raving lunatic." A week later, the then-23-year-old got his medical marijuana license.

The new, natural medication soothed his withdrawal symptoms as he weaned himself from the drugs his body had become so reliant on. By the time he was 25, he was off of all of them. His panic attacks became less frequent—dropping to one a month, then one every six months, until they ceased altogether. As of this writing, it had been three years since his last attack. He now medicates daily with a vaporizer pen, preferring sativa hybrids for his needs.

His new panic-attack-free life took some getting used to. "When you have panic attacks, you are a slave to your panic attacks," Alexei says. Suddenly, he was free to move about in the world and experience life in ways he couldn't imagine when he was shut in his room, riding the relentless currents of his anxiety.

"I remember going out to a coffee shop for the first time and sitting with a friend," he says. "I was having coffee and

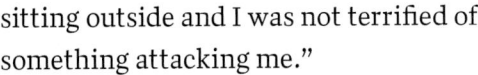

sitting outside and I was not terrified of something attacking me."

Triggers still pepper his surroundings, threatening to reawaken his demons, but he is able to cope with and manage them.

"If I can take my vape pen and vape quickly, I'm out of whatever dysfunction is going on with me really quickly," he says.

Occasionally, if a certain smell wafts his way, or the lighting in a room feels uncomfortably familiar, he will flash back to a scene that unfolded years ago in that Utah treatment center. But these dark moments of déjà vu are no longer followed by a crippling panic attack; he simply takes a pull on his vaporizer pen, and keeps moving on.

COMPARING SIDE EFFECTS

 COMPARING SIDE EFFECTS: Like any medicine, cannabis has side effects in addition to the treatment of a specific illness. Most notably, smoking or ingesting cannabis with moderate-to-high THC levels causes a user to feel high, or stoned, which can result in euphoric feelings and can affect short-term memory, concentration, sensory perception and coordination. Marijuana may also cause paranoia, anxiety and fear in some users, but cannot cause death by overdose. By comparison, pharmaceutical drugs commonly prescribed for depression and other mental disorders have a raft of potential side effects. For example:

 **• KLONOPIN (CLONAZEPAM)** is a benzodiazepine with numerous common side effects, including weakness, headaches, body pain, breathing trouble, depression, sleep disturbances, diarrhea, constipation, and blurred vision. Klonopin users can also experience confusion, hallucinations and exhibit unusual risk-taking behavior. The drug has serious habit-forming potential and can lead to suicidal thoughts. Overdoses can be fatal.

 • SEROQUEL (QUETIAPINE) is a psychotropic medication with its own array of side effects. People who take Seroquel sometimes deal with mood or behavior changes, chills, cold sweats, confusion, upset stomach, nausea, vomiting, dizziness, drowsiness and more. For older people with dementia, it can provoke heart failure and stroke. It can also create fetal health problems for pregnant women and can pass through breast milk into a nursing baby. Young people who take Seroquel sometimes have suicidal thoughts, and overdoses are potentially fatal.

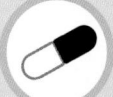 **• ZOLOFT (SERTRALINE)** is a selective serotonin reuptake inhibitor commonly prescribed for depression. Among other side effects are sleepiness, nervousness, insomnia, dizziness, nausea, headache, diarrhea, constipation and stomach pain. Some people experience aggressive reactions, paranoia, hallucination and psychotic disorders, and it can also cause various forms of sexual dysfunction. Zoloft has been known to provoke suicidal thoughts in users, particularly teenagers. Overdoses can be fatal.

Sources: Rxlist.com, NORML, Live Science, Drugs.com.

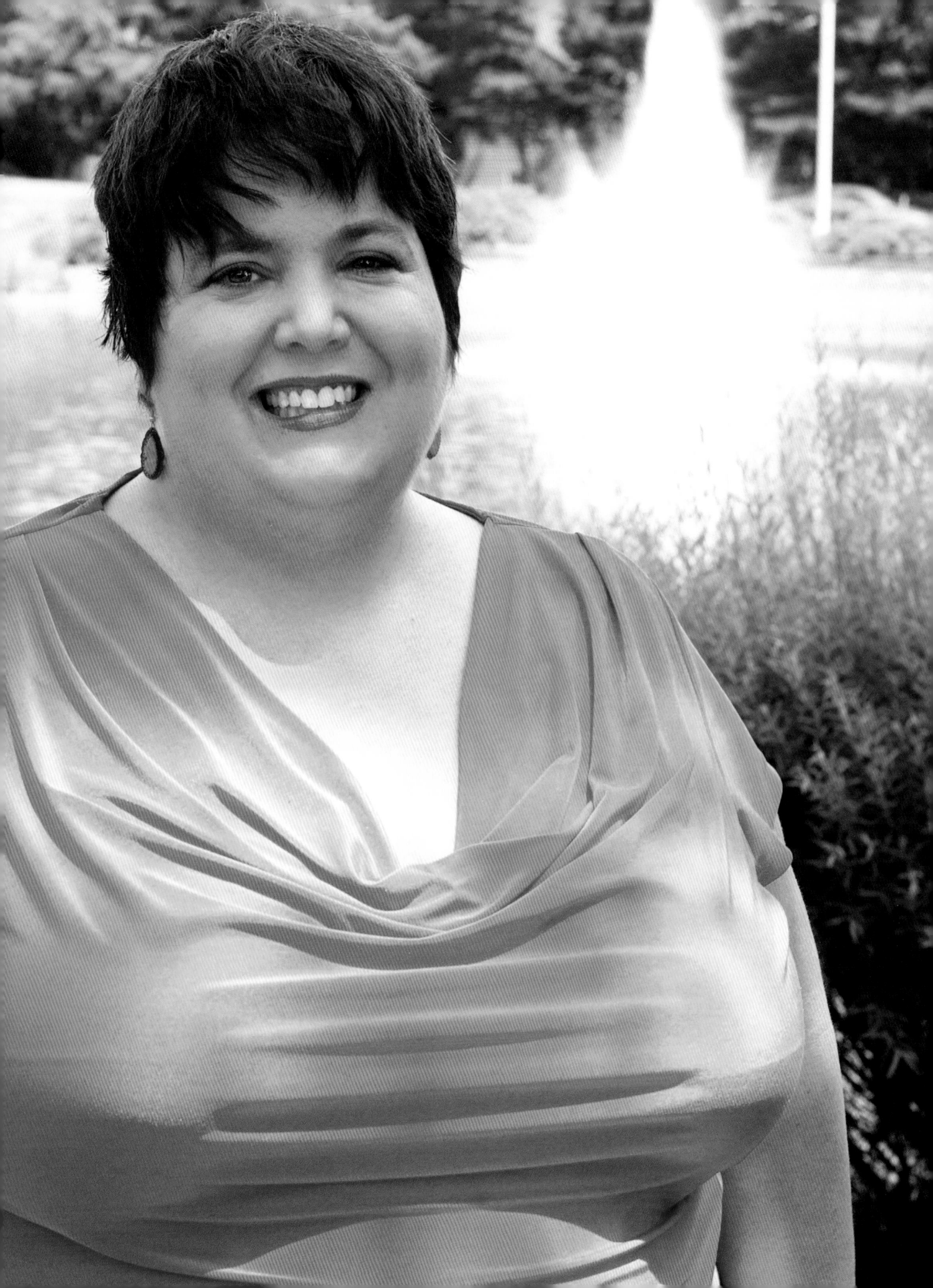

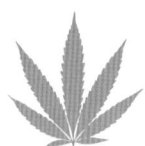

AMY ECHOLS

Age 41 / Lupus, Hashimoto's disease, Central Nervous System Vasculitis / Beaverton, Oregon

One day early in 2015, Amy Echols sat in her walker in the corner of a dance studio, watching her husband Johnathan lead a Zumba class. It seemed like any other class in recent years, with Amy relegated to the sidelines by her severe health issues, her own passion for teaching Zumba long since stifled.

But when the familiar opening notes of the closing number—"Careless Whisper," a Bachata-style song by the Latin music band Grupo Extra—came over the speakers, an urge came over Amy.

"I can do this," she thought.

She rose from her post in the corner and joined her husband at the front of the room. Through a veil of joyful tears, the couple led the last dance together, side-by-side. It was an emotional triumph for Amy, and a turning point in her recovery from a years-long battle with several devastating diseases.

"He turned off the music afterward and students came up and grabbed me," Amy says.

TINCTURE: Cannabis tinctures are made by soaking dried cannabis in alcohol, which extracts the THC and creates a liquid that preserves the psychoactive and medicinal properties of the original plant. Tinctures are taken orally or placed under the tongue and take effect relatively quickly. They are popular among patients who don't like to smoke or cannot smoke cannabis.

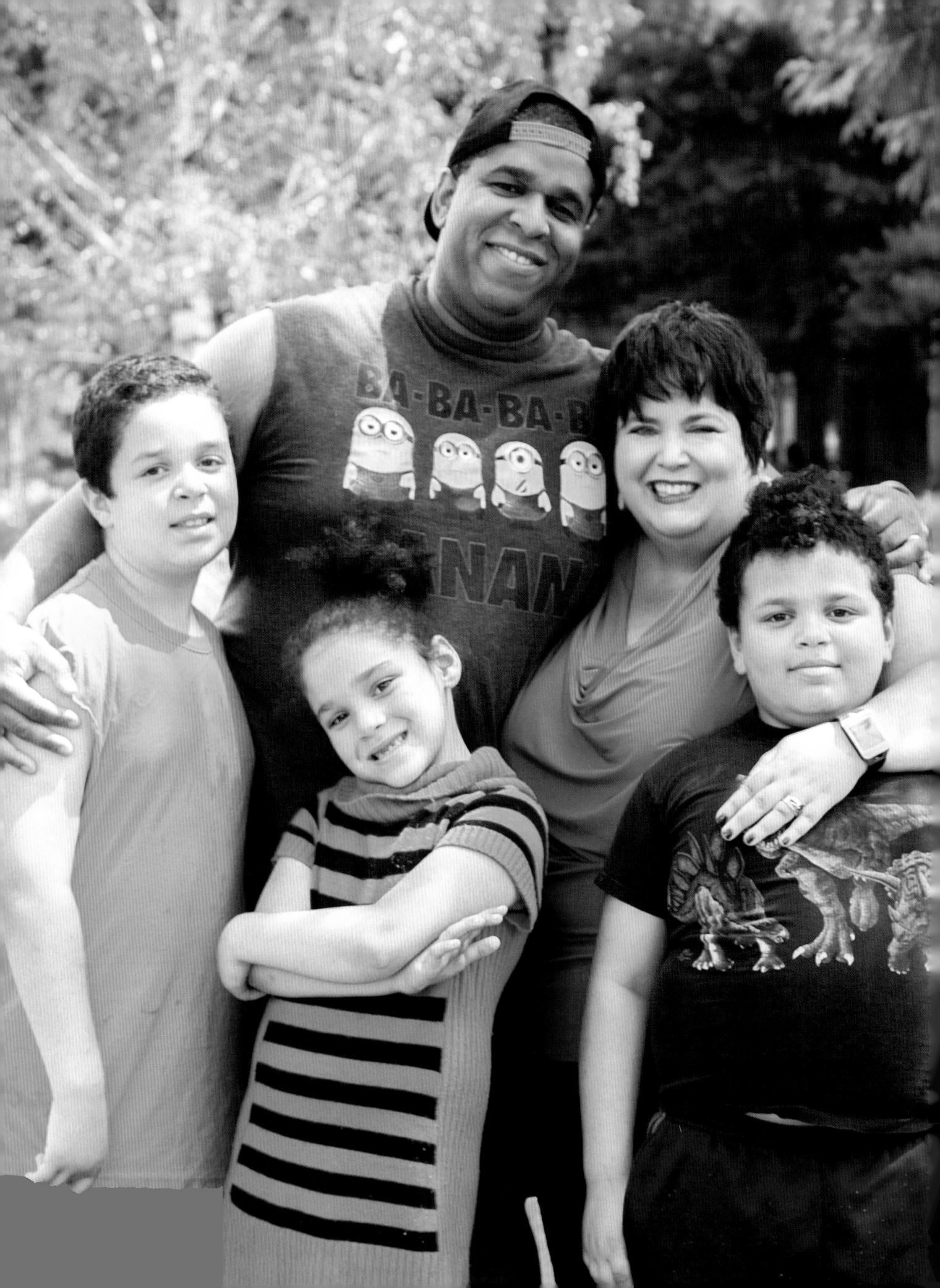

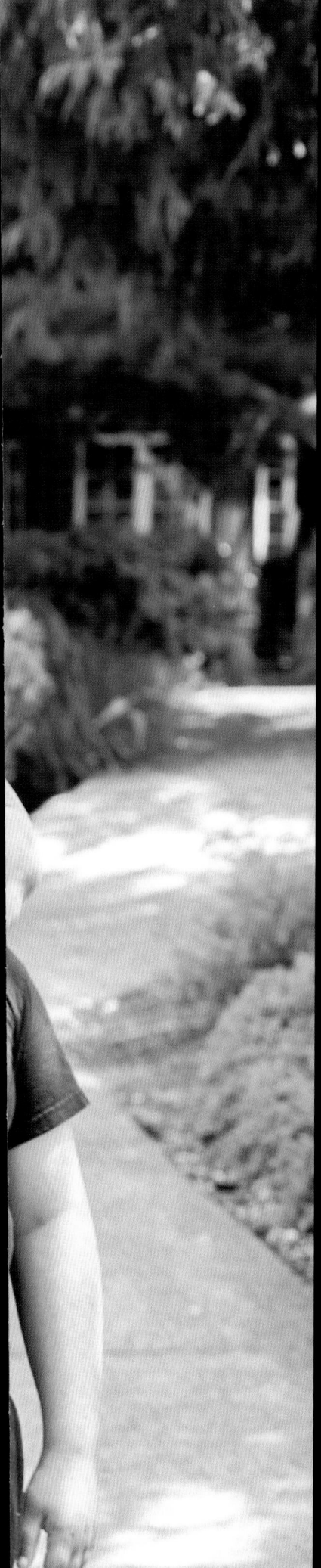

"IF I'D LET MY FEARS OF WEIGHT GAIN AND BEING STONED KEEP ME FROM [USING CANNABIS], I'D DEFINITELY BE HEAVIER THAN I AM NOW AND I MIGHT BE DEAD. AND INSTEAD, I'M PLAYING WITH MY KIDS . . . I'M OUT AND ABOUT, AND I'M LIVING LIFE."

The duo became certified Zumba instructors together after the birth of their youngest child, Rebecca, in 2008. But Amy's health, dictated by multiple autoimmune diseases, took a sudden turn for the worse in late 2010.

"Within a few weeks I couldn't stand to be touched, and walking felt like stepping on melting glass shards," Amy recalls. She later learned that it was a Lupus flare that hit her with this relentless, debilitating pain.

While it wasn't her first period of incapacitation at the hands of her conditions, it was the worst. During an eight-year struggle through 13 failed pregnancies (fortunately punctuated with the births of her three children in 2004, 2006 and 2008), Amy was diagnosed with Hashimoto's, a disease in which the immune system attacks the thyroid.

Her water broke when she was 26 weeks pregnant with Rebecca, kicking off a 57-day stint in the hospital and, once at home, months in bed, where she cried and prayed for things to improve. And they did—long enough for the Echols to became Zumba teachers. However, the longtime tap and tango dancer was eventually back in bed, angry and helpless, feeling like a shadow of her former self.

"When it got to the point that I couldn't dance, the depression was horrendous," she says.

In 2012, her doctors added Lupus and central nervous system vasculitis to her roster of diagnoses. The latter is a rare and hard-to-diagnose disorder that manifested for Amy as small strokes and loss of balance.

She was taking 26 different medications a day at a cost of $500 a month. "It was to the point where we had to use a laundry bag to bring my medicines home," she says. There was morphine for pain, and drugs for the Lupus, Hashimoto's, seizures, muscle spasms, depression, and fibromyalgia, "and then a bunch of rotating crap to try to counteract the side effects from those main ones," Amy adds.

"I was still in constant pain, still seizing, not sleeping, fighting anxiety," she says. "I just felt crappier with the side effects of the meds on top of everything else."

When her doctor ("bless his heart," she says) suggested that she consider cannabis, she rebuked the idea.

"I said 'No way! Not weed!'" she recalls. "I was raised in that 'Just Say No' era, and thought [people who use cannabis] are stoners and they sleep all day and eat munchies, and that I'd gain all this weight."

Her husband, who was also anti-cannabis up to that point, broke down in tears and asked her to at least try it. "What do we have to lose?" he pleaded.

"Within the first three months I lost 30 pounds," she says. "I was playing with my kids. For the first time in five years I walked down the stairs without a cane."

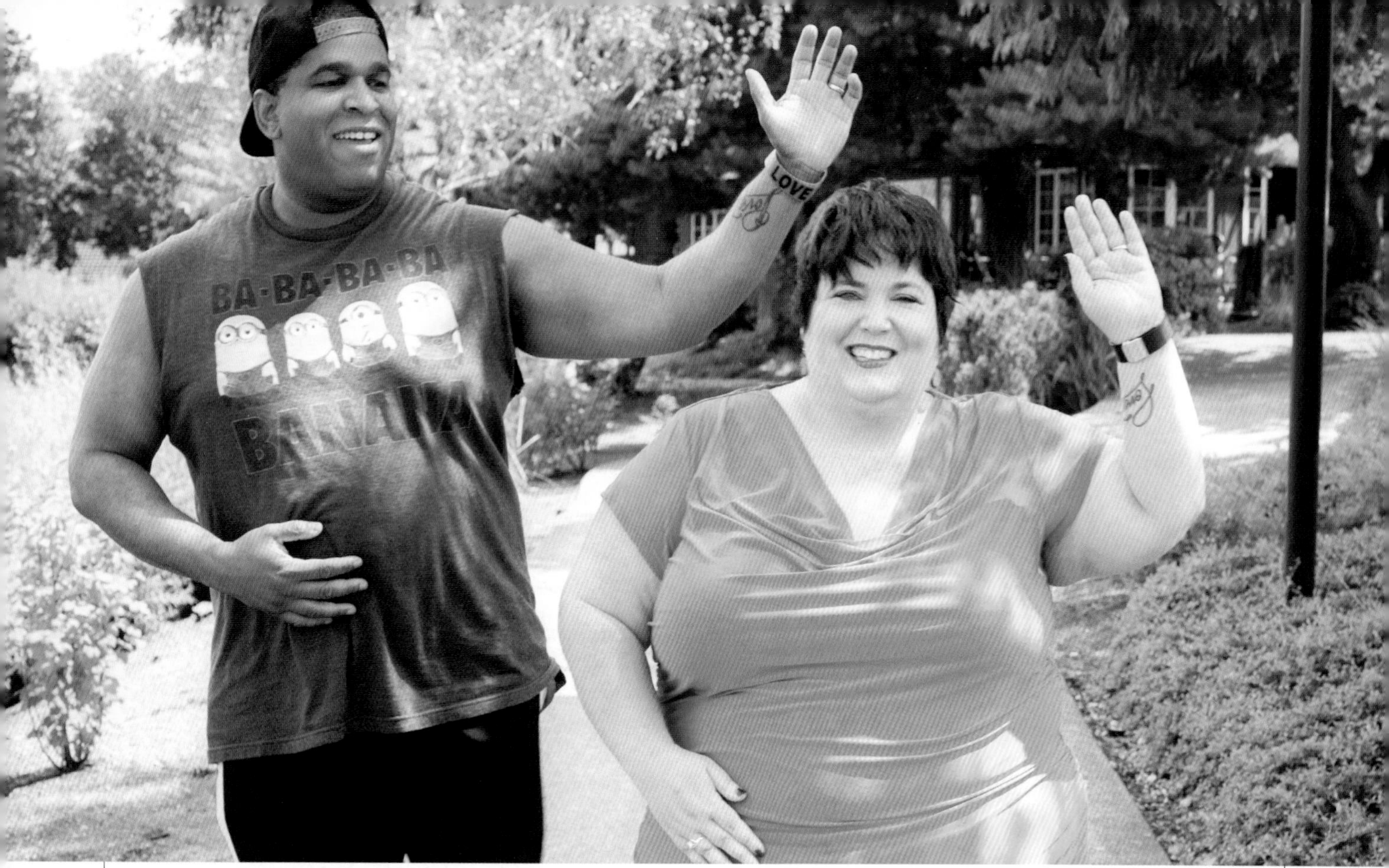

Two-dozen pharmaceuticals have been replaced with a cannabis tincture, a capsule at bedtime, and occasional use of a vaporizer. For the first time in her memory, she is sleeping seven hours a night, instead of her usual three.

"Today," Amy says, speaking one year and 89 lost pounds later, "I've done four loads of laundry, vacuumed, taken the kids to school—I never thought I'd be able to do that again, and all because of this plant. It's sad the misconceptions people have, and I had, about what this plant would do. If I'd let my fears of weight gain and being stoned keep me from it, I'd definitely be heavier than I am now and I might be dead. And instead, I'm playing with my kids, I'm out and about, and I'm living life."

And she's dancing again. She's helped her husband end his classes ever since that day, earlier this year, when she surprised everyone, herself included, by hopping up to do the Bachata.

"It's still a long road toward teaching a full class," she says, "but I have my eyes on the prize and I'm not about to quit."

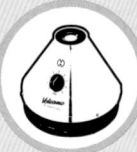

VAPORIZER: Vaporizers use heat to turn cannabis buds or other plant materials into a vapor that can be inhaled, as opposed to applying fire to the plant to create smoke. Many people prefer to use vaporizers because they don't create harmful toxins that accompany smoke, and therefore are suspected to be safer for your lungs. Vaporizing creates a near-instantaneous effect, similar to smoking, and it preserves more THC and other beneficial compounds than smoking does, so users need less marijuana to achieve the same results.

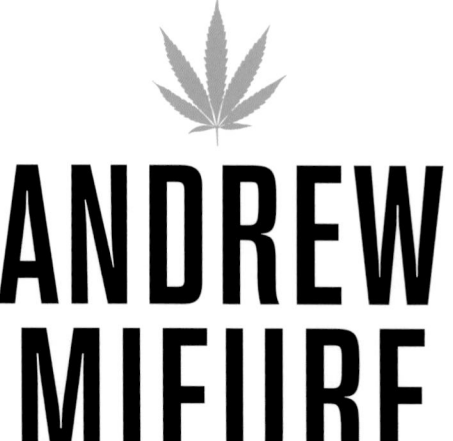

ANDREW MIEURE

Age 26 / **Anxiety** / Colorado Springs, Colorado

Last February, Andrew Mieure flew from Colorado, where he currently lives, to his home state of Ohio. It was uneventful.

And that made it remarkable.

The 26-year-old went to the airport, boarded the plane and sat through the flight without obsessing over everything that could go wrong. He didn't fixate on death, or have a panic attack. And he didn't have to numb himself with Xanax to make the journey possible. This was unimaginable to Andrew just a few years earlier—before he began using cannabis for his anxiety. Flying was the greatest of his many fears; fears so crippling that he often didn't venture outside or, for that matter, far from his bed.

"There would be times where I'd be laying in bed, not wanting to get up because I was afraid something was going to hurt me," says Andrew, whose symptoms developed when he was 20, just as they had for several of his relatives. "I'd lay in bed and my heart would be pounding, and I'd count my heartbeats to make sure it was beating correctly, because I wasn't sure it was."

The tentacles of his disorder wound their way around him out of the house, too, tightening their insidious grip while he drove, or as he helped customers at Best Buy, where he worked.

"I'd be driving to work and it felt like the car was closing in on me. Sometimes I'd have to stay only in the right lane, because if I was in the middle or left [lanes] I wouldn't be able to pull off the road just in case," he says. "At work, I'd be talking to clients and I'd get hot and cold sweats and a numbing, tingling feeling in my face."

A doctor put him on Xanax and Zoloft, which seemed to help, even if he felt a bit drunk. "I let life come and go without any passing thought," he says. "I didn't have any feeling toward anything."

Within a few months of taking the medications, he realized he didn't feel like himself anymore. His new reality was fuzzy and detached; his interactions with others were off kilter—if someone was speaking to him, he'd stare and respond several seconds later.

"I started thinking to myself, 'what's worse, this or the anxiety?' I was scared of the anxiety so I kept taking the pills because that's what felt good in the moment," he says.

But as he built up a tolerance, the dosages went up and more side effects surfaced: shaky hands, poor memory, ghost sensations, erectile issues, and "brain zaps"—electric shocks in the brain that caused Tourette's-like facial tics and stuttering.

Perhaps worst of all, Andrew's appetite disappeared, shrinking him to a malnourished 108 pounds. His ribs were visible on his 5-foot-5 frame.

The collective burden of it all hit Andrew, then 23 years old, one night as he lay in the bath. Soaking in the hot water, he realized this was no way to live, and he began to wonder what would be the easiest and least painful way to end his life.

Suicidal thoughts were unlike him, especially because he witnessed and bore the pain his grandfather's suicide caused his family when he was 5. So the emotional low point served as a wakeup call. The next day, he heard his inner voice say, "Those thoughts are dangerous and you need to stop what you're doing and figure out something else because this isn't working."

After hearing about an appetite-spurring synthetic cannabis drug from his doctor, Andrew's curiosity was piqued. "Cannabis, huh?" he thought to himself.

Andrew grew up in a religious, conservative household in a small Ohio farming community where marijuana

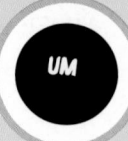

SYNTHETIC CANNABIS: There is a legal pharmaceutical synthetic cannabis product on the market called Marinol, or Dronabinol, which doctors can prescribe to AIDS and cancer patients to stimulate the appetite and control nausea. Marinol contains synthetic THC and is approved by the U.S. Food and Drug Administration. However, many practitioners still recommend natural cannabis products because synthetics such as Marinol are missing many of the other beneficial compounds, like CBD, that are found in marijuana. Not only do compounds like CBD have their own medicinal value, but they are also thought to act synergistically with THC to produce even more benefits, which are lost when the THC is produced in a lab in the absence of the other compounds. *Source: NORML, U.S. National Library of Medicine.*

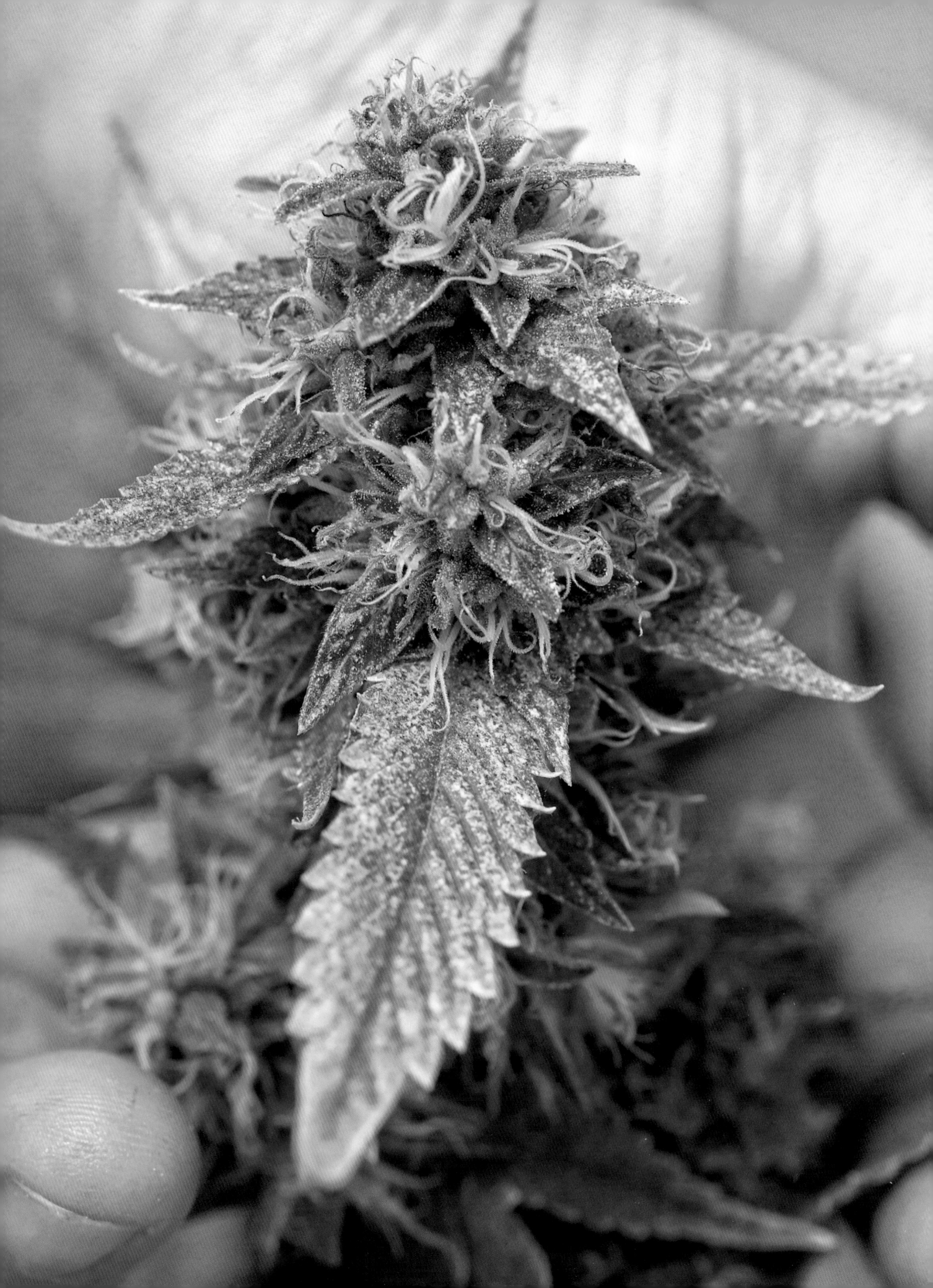

wasn't just a no-no; it was assumed to be as addicting and life ruining as heroin, which had indeed caused a sizable problem locally. He, even more so than many of his peers, was staunchly anti-pot. The others in his small graduating class of 30 would be shocked that the boy who called pot smokers "worthless pieces of shit" in high school ever came around to the plant. But, after more than six months of research, Andrew believed it was worth a try, and worked up the courage to ask a friend to enable a test run.

"I smoked it and I was sitting there, very calm, and I got really hungry," he says. "I started gorging on everything I could find. It felt good to feel hungry again. As I was coming down, I asked 'is that all it is?' My friend said 'yes.' I had been demonizing something all these years and that was all it was. From that moment on I was convinced there was something to it."

"It got me eating again. It helped me go to bed at night. It improved my quality of life," says Andrew, who has used it ever since. "I started having less problems with anxiety."

Andrew's research led him to learn about high-CBD strains (breeds of cannabis with greater amounts of the non-psychoactive and medically effective cannabinoids called cannabidiol), which sounded especially promising for his issues. But in the black markets of Ohio, it was hard enough to buy weed, let alone anything of consistent quality or specialized medical strains or products. His life

"WITHOUT ANXIETY GETTING IN THE WAY OF EVERYTHING, I CAN GO OUT IN PUBLIC AND DO THINGS. I CAN GO PLACES I'D NEVER GO BEFORE. I CAN ENJOY LIFE."

was so thoroughly improved, already, that he didn't hesitate: he and his girlfriend moved to Colorado in the fall of 2014 so he could medicate legally, safely and properly. Since relocating, he's found even greater relief.

"I was a victim to the thoughts in my head," he says. "Now, the thoughts that used to come through my head just aren't there anymore. I feel like myself again. Without anxiety getting in the way of everything I can go out in public and do things. I can go places I'd never go before. I can enjoy life."

Now 120 pounds and feeling healthier than ever, Andrew is working at a cannabis dispensary in Colorado and reviews CBD-rich varieties on his YouTube channel, CBD Strain Reviews. He says cannabis gave him his life back, and he wants to pay that gift forward.

"I directly attribute the plant to helping to save my life," he says. "And if people gave it a chance, it could help save theirs, too."

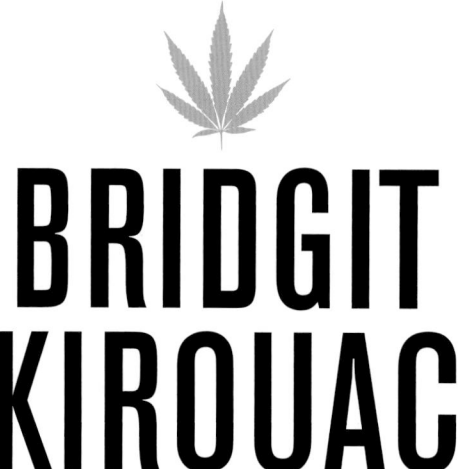

BRIDGIT KIROUAC

Age 53 / **Fibromyalgia, Psoriatic Arthritis** / Hobe Sound, Florida

By all outward appearances, Bridgit Kirouac seems like a normal 53-year-old woman.

Family, friends, and strangers, alike, are sometimes baffled by her use of a handicap placard, or by the cushion she carries tucked under her arm into restaurants. They shoot her funny looks or, worse, make judgmental remarks. *She looks fine, so why does she act so frail?*

Being misunderstood is a disheartening consequence of living with an invisible condition. Bridgit, like the five million other Americans who have fibromyalgia, has no perceptible manifestations of her suffering to conveniently signal to others how severe it is. There's no visible barometer of the toll her pain has taken on her body and mind—and that toll has been great.

Fibromyalgia is a cureless disorder believed to be rooted in how the brain processes pain signals; for its sufferers, pain sensations are amplified, resulting in chronic, widespread pain, sleep issues, fatigue and often depression.

Since her diagnosis in 1995, Bridgit has had to let go of the vestiges of her old life one by one. She said goodbye to beloved hobbies: no more skiing, ice-skating, canoeing, waterskiing, dancing, hiking, gardening, or aerobics. And, in 2011, when the occurrence of days on which she simply couldn't get out of bed became too frequent, her career in geographic information systems came to an early end.

"It's difficult to stay positive when you hurt all the time and when the things you enjoy doing keep slipping away

"THERE ARE REAL CRIMINALS OUT THERE THAT NEED THE ATTENTION OF LAW ENFORCEMENT. MY HUSBAND AND I ARE NOT AMONG THEM."

because you physically cannot do them anymore," she says.

Her professional and recreational routines long gone, now even basic things can be agonizing for Bridgit. Long drives or shopping excursions can land her in bed, recovering, for up to a week. She struggles with small tasks like holding the phone and typing on the computer. Squeezing toothpaste from the tube or opening the flip top on a bottle of ketchup causes excruciating pain. Even the sensation of clothing on her skin can be too much to bear.

"It's not just the feeling awful," she says, "it's the knowing that this is what you have to look forward to every day for the rest of your life—having no light at the end of the tunnel."

Bridgit has been riding a merry-go-round of pharmaceuticals for decades now in an attempt to manager the disorder.

"I can't even remember all the medications and 'therapies' that were tried on me," she says, rattling off a laundry list of the treatments she can recall: "a plethora of NSAIDS [nonsteroidal anti-inflammatory drugs], muscle relaxants, antidepressants, opiate medications including Oxycontin and fentanyl patches, thyroid medication, topical pain relievers, Lyrica, gabapentin, biofeedback, physical therapy, occupational therapy, pool therapy, massage therapy, chiropractic, psychotherapy, magnets, steroid injections, spinal surgery ... "

None of the drugs got her off the merry-go-round, nor slowed the ride down. Around and around she went without any sign of stopping, gaining long-term side effects like gastritis, hearing loss and vision problems. The most helpful treatments she has found to date are warm-water pool therapy, massage and medical cannabis. The latter has improved her wellbeing in myriad ways and curbed the onslaught of adverse prescriptions. It soothes her nausea, headaches, and inflammation, and, perhaps most importantly, it helps her sleep when used in conjunction with her prescriptions.

"Cannabis is a necessity," she says. "A hallmark of fibromyalgia is sleep disruption and non-restorative sleep. Because fibromyalgia also involves chronic widespread pain, sleep is critical. Without rest, there is no capacity whatsoever to deal with the pain."

As for the pain itself, cannabis does not lessen it, per se. Rather, it has the crucial effect of making it tolerable.

"Cannabis, like opiates, does not make the pain go away so much as it allows one to not dwell on the pain and be consumed by it," Bridgit says. "It allows me to be distracted from my pain without the terrible side effects associated with opiates, like hearing loss and severe constipation. It does not require me to take other medications to counteract its side effects, which are much more benign. I just drink a lot of water."

"For me, the unpleasant side effects of cannabis—dry mouth, red eyes—are much easier to deal with than the unpleasant side effects of most of the medications I have been prescribed, some of which have been pretty extreme and don't necessarily go away when you stop the medication," she adds.

Medicating with cannabis was easy when Bridgit and her husband, David, lived in Maine, which has had a medical marijuana law on the books since 1999. She secured a recommendation from a doctor, who wrote it for her pain and also for lingering PTSD from childhood sexual abuse, and began to grow marijuana as a patient.

In 2012, the Kirouacs decided to migrate to the small coastal hamlet of Hobe Sound, Florida, where the tropical climate eases some of Bridgit's discomfort. The Sunshine State was poised to legalize medical marijuana, or so the couple thought. Their disappointment was echoed throughout the state when the Florida Right to Medical Marijuana Initiative fell 3 percent short of the necessary 60 percent majority approval in the November 2014 election.

"I had hoped that by the time what medicine I had canned [as tinctures] in Maine ran out, Florida would have a medical marijuana law," Bridgit says.

But when the last mason jar of honey-like tincture ran dry, Florida was no closer. And without legal avenues or any local friends or acquaintances in her new state to obtain it from, Bridgit set up a self-contained tent in her garage and began growing it herself.

In May 2014, half a dozen SWAT officers raided the Kirouacs' home, slashing the growing tent, smashing the grow lights, and seizing the plants and all of her ready-to-use cannabis medicines throughout the house. The couple was handcuffed and questioned, first in their home and then at the agents' offices, before being taken to the county jail and processed—by which time Bridgit was "up around a nine on a one-to-10 pain scale." A few hours later they posted bail and took a cab home. But the legal troubles had only just begun.

Her husband works in another county, and the couple would be in danger of losing their home if he could not keep his job. For this reason—and because he doesn't use cannabis and could therefore comply with drug-free stipulations—he decided to accept a tendered plea of 12 months' probation.

"He has been forced to pay not only a fine and court costs, but for a substance-abuse evaluation, substance-abuse classes—remember, he does not use cannabis or any other illegal drug—and a supervision fee for every month that he's on probation," Bridgit explains.

Bridgit, however, relies on cannabis to function, and consequently decided to fight the felony possession and cultivation charges levied against her based on the legal doctrine of "medical necessity." As of this writing, Bridgit was awaiting a midsummer status hearing.

"There are real criminals out there that need the attention of law enforcement," she says. "My husband and I are not among them."

Meanwhile, her health took a turn for the worse. She was diagnosed with Psoriatic Arthritis around the time of the raid and began a new cycle of pharmaceuticals to address it. One dose of the first, methotrexate, caused a debilitating fibromyalgia flare up that knocked her out for the entire summer.

"Once I started to feel a little better from that, I did a trial of Otezla," she explains. "Two months of feeling sick to my stomach all the time, and it really aggravated my vertigo. So we discontinued it, gave myself a little time for my stomach to feel better, then started Enbrel, an injection I had to give myself once a week. This caused some pretty pronounced injection-site reactions, left me feeling quite depressed and caused abdominal pain. And it had no effect on my pain and inflammation. So now I'm on Humira."

"Thus far," she adds, "I have used cannabis to counteract the side effects of all of these medications, none of which have helped at all."

Through it all, she tries to stay positive. "Without cannabis I would have no quality of life," she says. "My pain would so consume my consciousness that I would spend every ounce of energy I have, which isn't much, coping with it."

Instead, she does the laundry and grocery shops, and enjoys reading books on her tablet. On a good day, she might walk the dog, tread water at the pool or have lunch with a friend.

"The list of things I can't do is much, much, longer," she says, "but I choose to focus on what I still can do, rather than on what I can't."

FIBROMYALGIA: Fibromyalgia is a disease that causes fatigue and musculoskeletal pain, particularly in the neck, spine, shoulders and hips. There is no known cure, but many patients find marijuana helps relieve pain and other symptoms. A 2014 online survey sponsored by the National Pain Foundation found that patients said medical marijuana was better at treating fibromyalgia symptoms than FDA-approved drugs, with 62 percent of respondents saying it was "very effective." *Sources: National Pain Report, NORML*

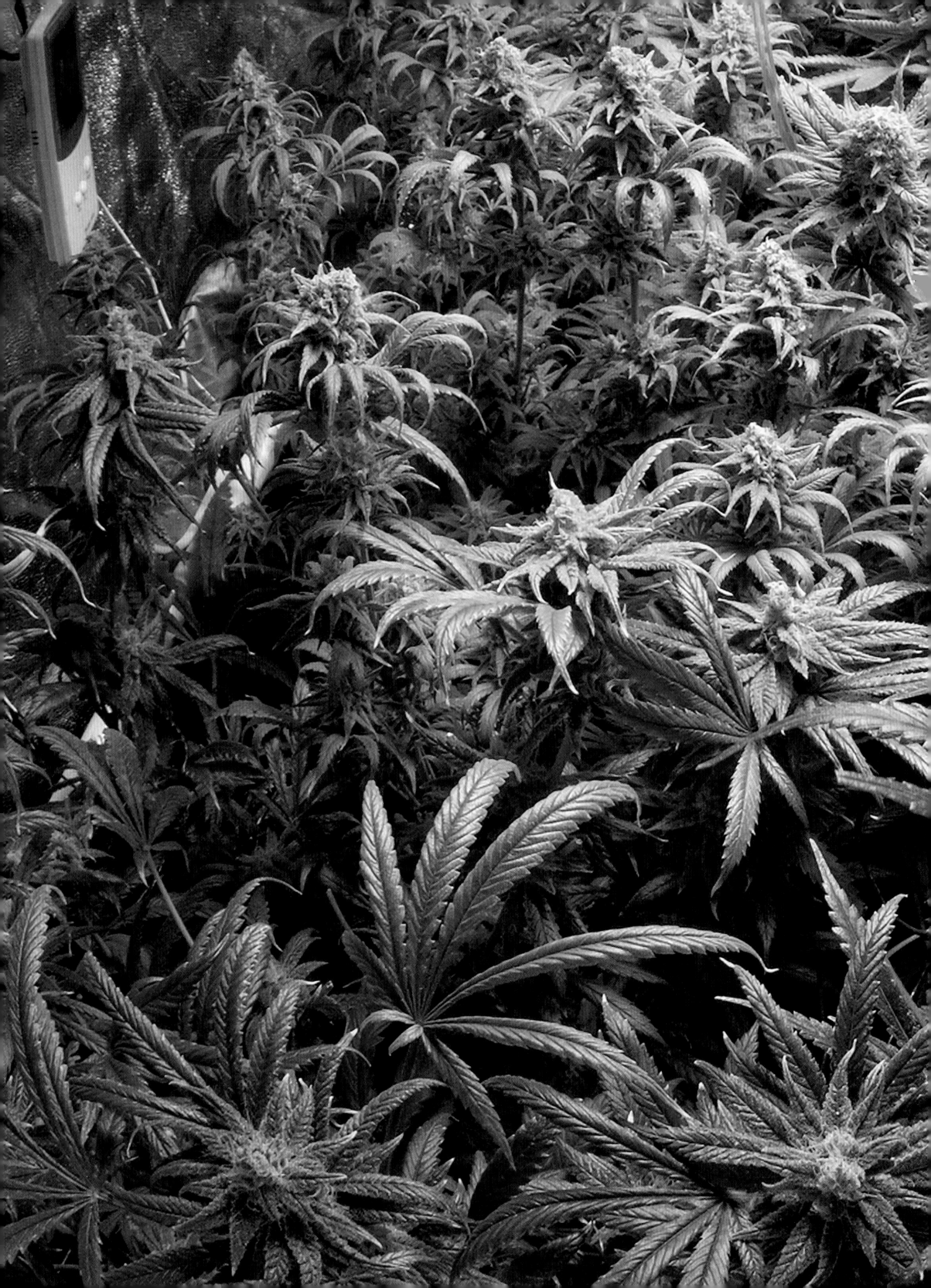

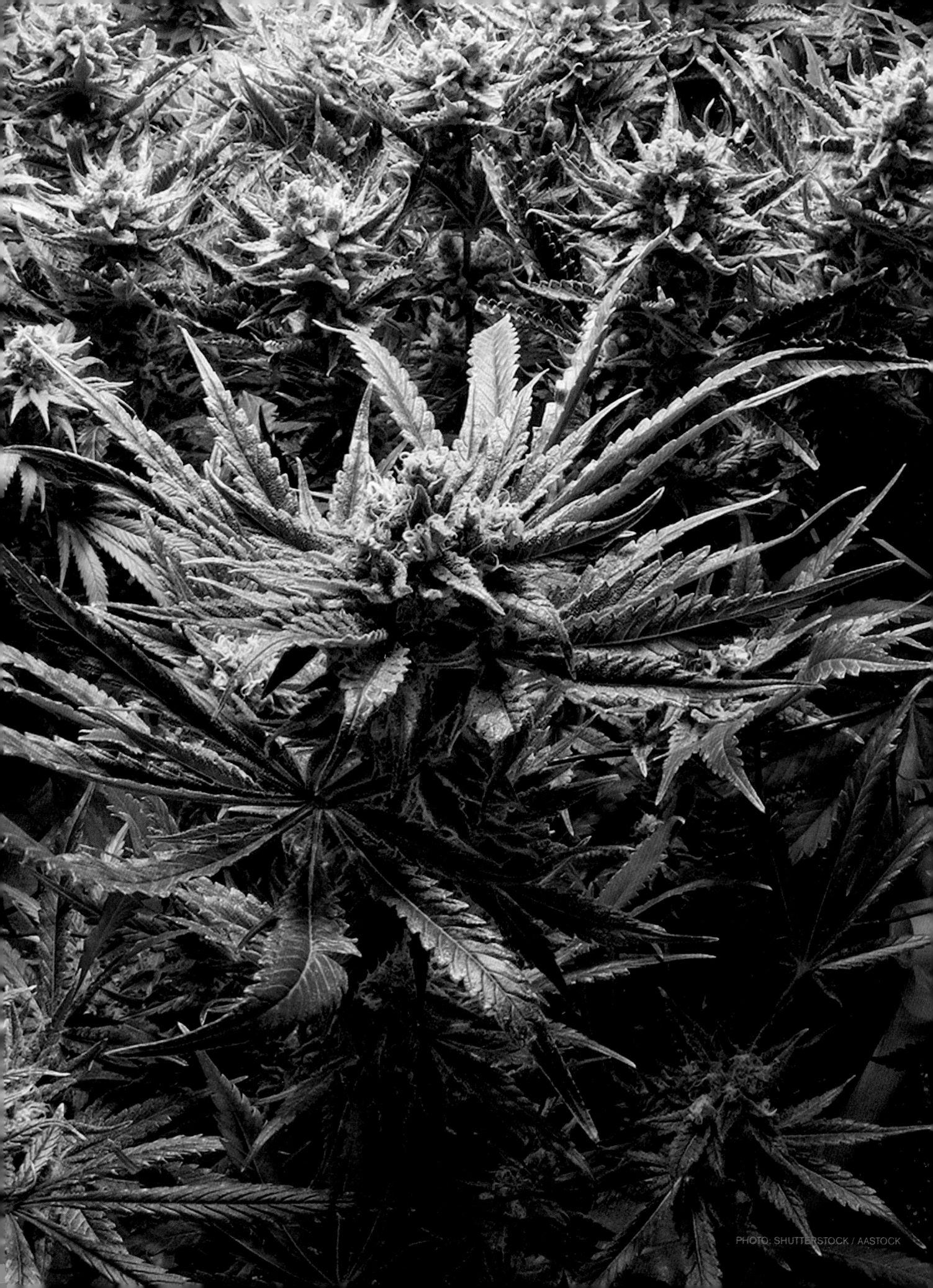

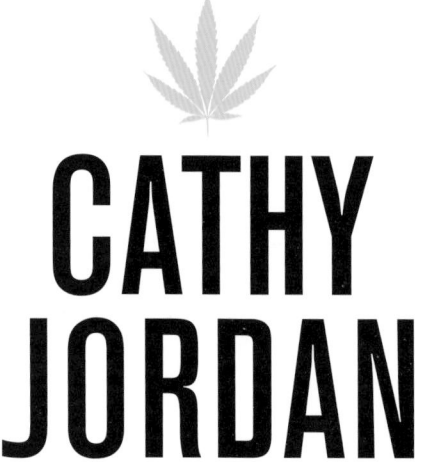

CATHY JORDAN

Age 64 / **Lou Gehrig's disease** / Parrish, Florida

There were times in Cathy Jordan's fight for the legalization of medical marijuana when she was too tired and too weak to hold the phone. Her husband, Bob, watched her hold back tears, set the phone on the table, lay her head down against it, and carry on making calls.

"She'd call everyone who would listen," Bob says, "and finally people did start to listen."

Today, Cathy is an in-demand spokesperson for medicinal cannabis. She's featured in news articles and television programs, and can often be found on the frontlines at demonstrations, hearings and conferences. It's a taxing undertaking for someone living with Lou Gehrig's disease, or ALS, and the diminished capabilities it entails. But she's determined to exert her remaining energy to spread the word that cannabis can save lives.

After all, she would know: she is living proof.

Cathy was diagnosed with ALS in 1986, four years into her marriage to Bob, with whom she raised three children. They lived in Newcastle, Delaware, where Bob worked in a steel mill. Cathy was a hairdresser by day and tended bar by night. "Life was good," says Bob.

The first sign that something was wrong were Cathy's hands. Early in 1986, she began having trouble getting her fingers out of the handles on her haircutting scissors. A few months and a series of painful tests and surgeries later, a neurologist confirmed the ALS diagnosis and said she would be lucky to live five more years.

The news was unfathomable.

"She's still healthy looking, and still doing hair, and still bartending, and they say she only has three to five years to live," Bob says. "Devastating is not the correct word. It was beyond devastating. At first you don't believe it."

But once it takes hold, ALS moves fast. What often begins as muscle weakness and stiffness snowballs into paralysis and deterioration of the muscles, including, eventually, the muscles in charge of swallowing, speaking and breathing. The average life expectancy of a person with ALS is two to five years after diagnosis, according to the ALS Association.

Cathy soon spent her days under a pile of blankets on the couch, immobile from pain, barely able to eat, and zombie-like from the host of prescriptions she was on.

In a video titled "Surviving ALS #2: Back to 1986"—one of several powerful installments about Cathy's journey that can be found on her YouTube channel, youtube.com/SurvivingALS—Bob sits beside Cathy on a tan couch, wiping tears from his cheeks with a crumpled tissue, as he relays what they were told to expect.

"'You're either going to choke to death, suffocate, or deteriorate down to nothing,'" he recalls doctors saying. "'Get your affairs in order—you've got three to five years to live and it's just going to keep getting worse.'"

2 TO 5 YEARS

THE AVERAGE LIFE EXPECTANCY AFTER AN ALS DIAGNOSIS, ACCORDING TO THE ALS ASSOCIATION.

The scene cuts away to a home video with a time stamp of Dec. 31, 1988—a celebration for Cathy's 38th birthday. Through a doorway, the viewer sees her in the kitchen, framed by the multicolor glow of a strand of Christmas lights. Her blonde hair hangs loose above the shoulders of her baggy grey sweatshirt.

A few frames later, the video captures a toast made in Cathy's honor. She looks down at her cup and shakes with little sobs. Unbeknownst to anyone else at the time, Cathy had decided to kill herself.

"This will be my last birthday," she thought.

As predicted by her doctors, the disease was progressing quickly. Her life and her spirit were becoming unfamiliar to her. And, as a fiercely independent woman, she could not bear the thought of becoming a burden to her family. Rather than allow ALS to take her as its victim, she elected to end her life on her terms. She covertly hoarded her muscle relaxers and arranged a trip to visit a friend in Florida, where she would swallow the pile of pills one night and never wake up.

She kept the decision from even her husband, who encouraged the trip because Cathy benefits from warmer climates.

"I thought it was for her to get out of the cold weather, but she was actually saving up her muscle relaxers to commit suicide," Bob explains via speakerphone,

"I ALWAYS SAY THAT THE PHARMACEUTICALS KILLED MY SPIRIT AND CANNABIS BROUGHT MY SPIRIT BACK."

pausing occasionally when Cathy interjects, listening patiently to her distorted speech and then repeating her comments for my understanding. "We'd be sitting down and all of a sudden she'd start choking. Me and my son, we'd run over and move her arms and massage her neck to stop her from choking. She says that the fear she saw in us—that's when she knew that she was not going to go out that way."

In Florida, as Cathy's days grew numbered, she and a friend went to Bradenton Beach to smoke a joint.

Suddenly, as Cathy teetered on the verge of suicide, something smaller and lighter than a felt-tip pen pushed her back to safety. And back to life. Amongst the crash of waves and gusts of salty air, Cathy felt her unrelenting disease pause. For the first time in years, she felt fine— better than fine. Back at her friend's house, she devoured Ritz crackers slath-

ered in peanut butter and jelly. She couldn't remember the last time she'd been this hungry or that food had tasted this good.

In the YouTube video, Cathy relays this story 20 years later, parked in her wheelchair on the wooden walkway that leads down to Bradenton Beach. Her speech is belabored and choppy—a trademark of ALS—but she describes the experience with an unfading smile.

"I always say that the pharmaceuticals killed my spirit," Cathy says, the same auspicious stretch of sand behind her, "and cannabis brought my spirit back."

She extended her stay by three weeks and, when it was finally time to fly home to Delaware, she put a half-ounce of Myakka Gold—the locally grown marijuana strain she'd been smoking—in a glass cigar vile, corked it, and hid it between her breasts. In the video, the couple laughs as Bob remembers his

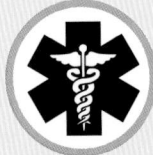

MEDICAL NECESSITY: In states where medical marijuana is not legal, patients who are prosecuted for possessing or consuming cannabis may argue in court that their use of the substance is medically necessary. A defendant making this claim would acknowledge that he or she broke the law, but argue that cannabis use was the "lesser evil" compared to succumbing to a debilitating illness. Medical necessity arguments need to show that there is no legal alternative treatment for the medical condition in question, and require testimony from a medical expert. *Source: NORML.org.*

reaction when Cathy revealed her stowaway goods back in Delaware: "Jesus Christ! You'll get busted for smuggling! What in the hell is the matter with you? You crazy?"

"They all thought I was insane," Cathy adds.

But Bob's alarm about the marijuana was nothing compared to his disbelief over Cathy's 180-degree improvement.

"The best way I can explain it is that the woman I sent to Florida was dying," he says, "and the woman who came home from Florida was living."

"I said, OK if you think [marijuana] will make you feel better I'll go along with it," he goes on. "I didn't believe her. She had three to five years to live, so I was trying to be understanding about it. But lo and behold, she started getting better. She was walking better, eating better, not choking, talking better."

Her doctor was less supportive. When Cathy mentioned the cannabis use to him, he turned to Bob as if she weren't there, looked him in the eye, and suggested he consider putting her in a psychiatric hospital. Echoes of "Just Say No" were still ringing out across the country as the '90s began, and ALS, as far as her doctors were concerned, was a death sentence. Nothing, especially not a Cheech and Chong-endorsed "gateway drug," was going to change that for her.

Bob lost his job around this time, when the steel mill where he worked

5,600

THE NUMBER OF AMERICANS DIAGNOSED WITH ALS EACH YEAR.

closed, and their home went into foreclosure. The couple's friends in Florida offered to put them up until they could get back on their feet.

"I asked the doctor, 'Will warm weather be better for her?' He said, 'Absolutely.' I said 'OK, that's it. We're going. I ain't got nothing to lose,'" Bob recounts. "He said, 'Don't be fooled, though, she has one more year of mobility, maybe, and two more years bedridden, and then she'll suffocate and die.'"

The Jordans arrived in Florida on April Fools' Day 1991, and have lived there ever since. The first marijuana plant Bob grew for Cathy at their new home was ready for harvest a year later on Valentine's Day. He wrapped it in newspaper and brought it to her like a bouquet of roses.

"I stood before God and man and said 'in sickness and health,' and I meant it," Bob says of his commitment to Cathy. "It's not easy, but I know two things for absolute certain: one day I'm going to die, and if this situation were reversed, she'd be here with me."

Every morning, he makes Cathy a cup of hot coffee while she smokes a joint rolled with a sativa-dominant strain called Pure Power Plant. And then comes the coughing—the most significant benefit Cathy experiences from using cannabis.

"Most ALS patients choke to death or drown on their own saliva. They can't cough," Bob says, describing a device

ALS patients wear that simulates a cough by squeezing their lungs and pushing mucus out. "Every morning she smokes one to two joints and all that stuff comes out."

Early in their Florida days, Cathy recalls seeing a new neurologist who was the first of her many doctors to support—albeit vaguely—her self-medication.

"Can I ask you something?" the doctor said. "What are you doing? All my other patients are getting worse and you're staying the same."

"If you ask your assistant to leave I'll tell you," Cathy replied. The assistant left the room. "I smoke pot."

The doctor was already flabbergasted at the rate at which she'd slowed this swift disease; now he was stunned by the illegal remedy that she'd used to do so. Unable to discuss it further, he left her with this advice: "Don't tell another soul, but keep doing what you're doing."

Cathy's faint voice rises on the line: "He was my first possible believer."

"He was her first possible believer," Bob repeats into the phone.

It's been several decades since Cathy was supposed to die—a survival rate so rare for ALS that she has become something of "a unicorn," in Bob's words, to the medical community. Doctors swarm around her at conferences, eager to see the infamous ALS survivor with their own eyes.

Medical professionals are not the only ones baffled by Cathy. In 1995, Social Security sent a letter to the Jordans requesting that Cathy prove she was still alive. "She got a letter from Social Security because she outlived her expiration date," Bob says with a laugh. "They thought I had her buried in the backyard and was keeping her checks."

"There is no doubt she has ALS," Bob goes on. "She's in a wheelchair, she can't move her arms, she can't dress herself, and she can walk just a little bit. But she's mentally alert. It's taken years and years for that to happen, when it would have taken months."

The couple kept Cathy's cannabis use fairly quiet at first. Then, in 1995, a doctor said that her illegal drug use meant she would not be eligible for an ALS cure if one should ever surface.

The threat flipped a switch for Cathy: her voice might be hard to decipher, but

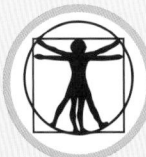

ALS: Amyotrophic lateral sclerosis, better known as ALS or Lou Gehrig's disease, is a neurodegenerative disease characterized by a hardening in the spinal cord that prevents messages from the brain from reaching the body. Cannabis can help protect the nerves that control body movement by stimulating the endocannabinoid system, as well as relieve symptoms of ALS. Studies have shown cannabis can delay motor impairment and prolong survival in animals, but non-anecdotal research on humans has been stymied by federal regulations. *Sources: ALS Association, Americans for Safe Access.*

"DON'T LET THE WHEELCHAIR FOOL YOU—SHE'S COURAGEOUS. WHEN WE GO TO TALLAHASSEE AND [LEGISLATORS] SEE THE WHEELCHAIR COMING, THEY TURN AROUND AND GO THE OTHER WAY." —BOB JORDAN

she wasn't going to stay silent any longer. She wanted to be heard.

Her first public speech was at the 1997 Hemp Fest in Tampa, kicking off the couple's nearly 20-year spree of activism. They're glad to report that they've seen attitudes about cannabis evolve in that time, but they lament that there is still a long way to go in their home state of Florida. Case in point: on Feb. 25, 2013, just two days after they appeared at the state capitol to lobby for The Cathy Jordan Medical Cannabis Act (a senate bill that would have legalized medical marijuana for qualified patients if it had passed), the Jordans' home was raided by law enforcement and Bob was hit with felony charges for the cultivation of 23 plants, the majority of which were tiny seedlings. Legal woes ensued, culminating in their receipt of "medical necessity" and the dismissal of the charges.

The affront only stoked the Jordans' fervor to return cannabis to its rightful place as a medicine that lessens suffering and, as Cathy shows, save lives. As of this writing, the Jordans await a jury trial for their consequential lawsuit against the sheriff. It's fueled by symbolic, rather than financial, motivations; the couple believes their case could set a precedent in Florida that would help all patients find long-awaited "protection under the law."

When asked what keeps her going through all of this, Cathy's voice is encumbered but her resolve rings clear: "I want to end the drug war."

The tenacious warrior wants to free the sick and dying who have been held captive as prisoners of this war. And she does it all from the confines of her rebelling body: she cannot scratch her own nose if it itches, yet she's become a nationally recognized activist and beacon of hope for the ALS community.

"If you ask Cathy what she wants, she wants it all and she wants it now," Bob says. "Don't let the wheelchair fool you—she's courageous. When we go to Tallahassee and [legislators] see the wheelchair coming, they turn around and go the other way."

"If a woman with ALS can accomplish what she's accomplished," he adds, "there is no excuse for anybody else."

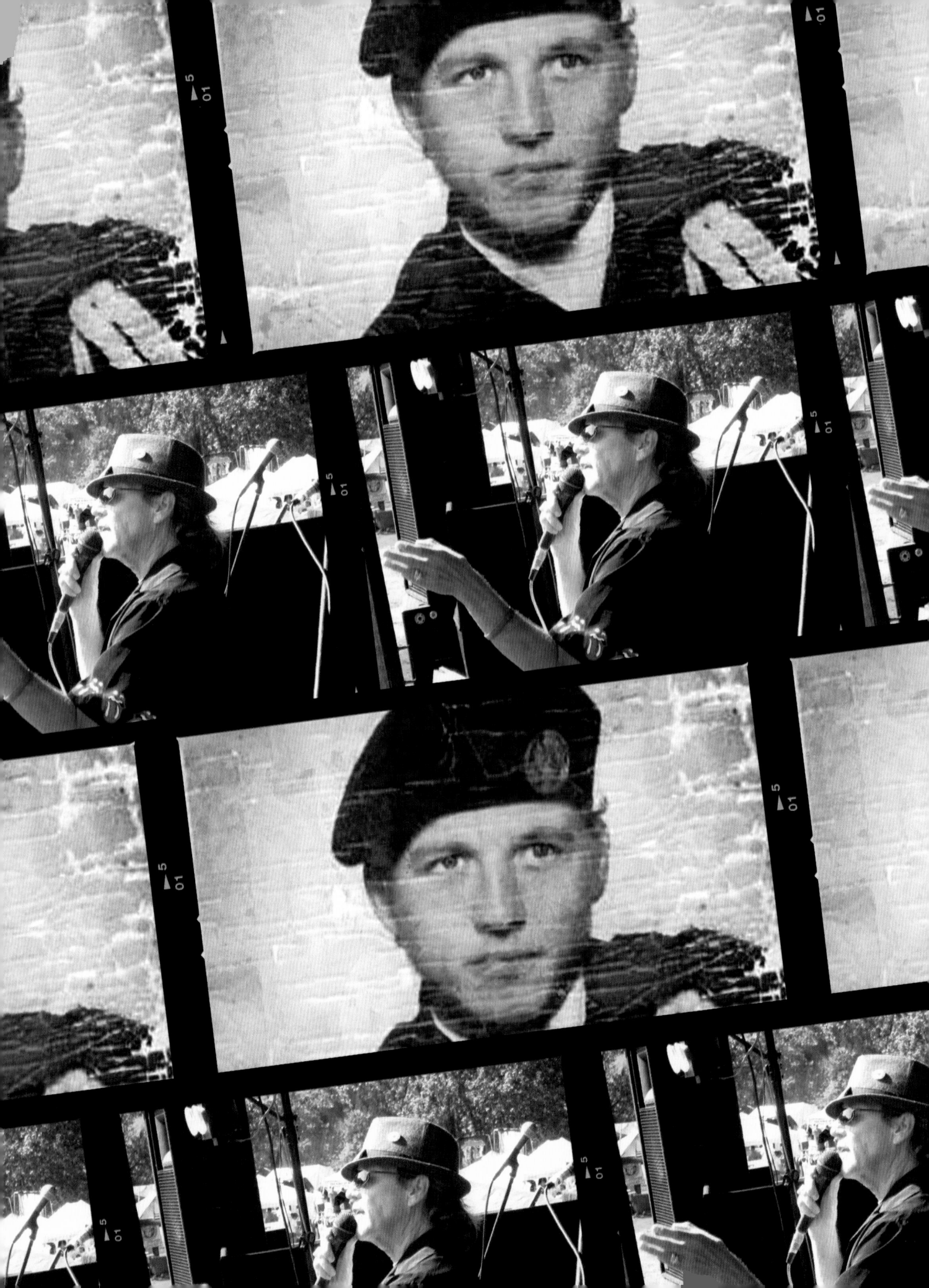

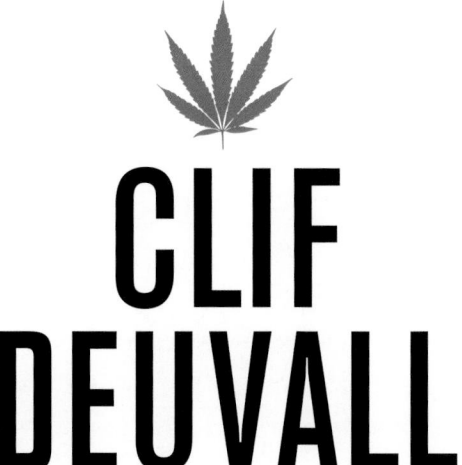

CLIF DEUVALL

Age 60 / **Intractable Neuropathic Pain** / Waco, Texas

Clif Deuvall has an eyeball for every occasion. For upbeat events, he might pop in a clear one with a rainbow prism, à la Pink Floyd's *Dark Side of the Moon*, or another orb that's awhirl with tie-dye. If he's feeling a bit more macabre, he may go the route of solid black with a grey iris. "It's sort of dead looking," he jokes.

For more serious matters, such as lobbying for medical marijuana at the Texas capitol, the disabled veteran and former high school teacher wears one of the realistic—and decidedly less interesting—glass eyes in his growing collection.

Clif lost his right eye in 2003 after decades of health issues stemming from his service in the Vietnam War, when he incurred brain lesions and neurologically rooted pain. The funkier of the glass eye replacements make him easy to spot at the many functions he attends as an activist—a role he's taken on since discovering cannabis to be the most effective treatment in his struggle with intractable neuropathic pain. The glass eyes are also a sober reminder of what he's been through.

When he spoke at Portland's Hempstalk Festival in 2013, Clif sported a brick-red eye with a white pupil and small green pot leaf in the center. Backstage, a passerby jumped back in fright at the sight of him. "Do I need to call the medics?" the man asked, staring at the crimson eye. Clif reassured him that it was fake.

It was a very similar moment, 10 years earlier, which made that glass eye necessary in the first place.

A VETERAN'S STRUGGLE

One morning in 1975, Clif awoke racked with pain and nausea. Looking around his quarters at the Yokota Air Base near Tokyo, he was startled to realize that he could barely see. It was like trying to gaze through a room full of smoke.

He was flown to a naval station that housed the nearest eye doctor, and was told he had glaucoma and was no longer qualified for duty. After being relocated to a stateside base in Albuquerque, New Mexico, Clif underwent operations on his eyes, as well as for injuries to his legs, before being discharged on a medical basis in 1978. In addition to the glaucoma diagnosis, he went on to suffer through decades of crippling widespread pain, nausea and headaches, without an answer as to what was the cause.

He was heavily medicated by the VA from 1975 on, but his disability level was low enough after returning to civilian life that he was able to pursue a career, first with Department of Defense contractors and later, after returning to school for a degree in education, as a social studies teacher. He excelled as an educator, earning a Texas Senate Teacher of the Year Commendation for his work at A.J. Moore Academy, where he taught AP-level government and economics.

He trudged through a series of operations on his knees, wrist and eyes, as his vision in the right eye shrunk to "a pinhole surrounded by darkness." Doctors maintained that he had glaucoma but could not discern which type. They sliced and diced the right eye with lasers and surgery, unintentionally spurring the organ to generate more and more blood vessels in attempt to heal itself—an increasingly agonizing build-up that came to a dramatic end one day in 2003 while Clif was lecturing to his students.

Clif felt a sharp pain in his eye but didn't think much of it until a student caught his attention and said that his eye was turning red. He rushed to his office and looked in the mirror. Blood was rising in his eye like water pouring into a glass.

"The pain was insurmountable," Clif says. When the eye was removed later that year, it became clear that Clif didn't have glaucoma like he'd been told for the last 28 years. The problem had been an injury all along—a revelation reinforced soon after by a neurologist who discovered five lesions splayed across the right hemisphere of Clif's brain, arranged in a blooming pattern that arched from front to back.

"No wonder you have a lot of pain," the doctor said. "Were you ever in an explosion?"

Clif's thoughts turned to a spring morning in Saigon in 1975. He'd been sitting in an aircraft on the tarmac when direct fire hit further down the line of planes. He sprang from his seat to help and was thrown 15 feet by the force of another blast. "I got shoved to the ground," he says, "but I really didn't feel like I got hurt."

"Well, that was probably what did it," the doctor replied, casting new clarity on Clif's ongoing maladies.

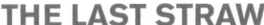

THE LAST STRAW

It was then that Clif was diagnosed with intractable neuropathic pain, an incurable pain disorder that targets the cardiovascular, hormone, and neurologic systems. Veterans Affairs reacted by "putting me on every kind of medication you can possibly imagine," Clif says. "They even had me on anti-psychotics at one point because they said it would help control the pain." From 2003 to 2005, Clif juggled as many as 16 prescriptions a day.

"In 2005 they took me off of everything and put me on methadone to try to control my pain, because of course that's the last straw," he says. "I was taking it three times a day. I went from being a commended educator of the year to 100-percent unemployable."

He dropped from 165 pounds to a frail 108 and felt his life slipping away with each pound: his job, his plans to pursue a doctoral degree, his quality of life all evaporated as he wasted away. The once-acclaimed educator was living in his bathrobe, barely able to put a sentence together, in a four-year methadone stupor that he can't remember.

"How much longer do I have to be on this drug regimen?" he asked his doctor, fed up. The answer terrified him: "For the rest of your life."

"The VA basically sent me home to live out the last few years of my life dependent on methadone," Clif says. But he had other plans for himself. After a spell of nasty withdrawals, he quit the methadone. He dove into research, ravenous for any option he had yet to try.

"I'd already been through the ringer with pharmaceuticals," he says. "I was looking at alternative medications and found out that cannabis was exactly what I needed." The results were immediate: lower pain levels, higher cognitive abilities, and the ability to live an active, engaged life once again. Today, he's down from five brain lesions to two.

"For over almost 30 years, every day I got up and the first thing I did was vomit," he says. "Every morning. Even when I was on pain medication I'd get sick. Now it's very rare. It's maybe twice a year when my pain levels get so high that I actually get sick."

The experience catapulted him into the world of advocacy: he founded a Waco chapter of the nonprofit marijuana lobbying organization NORML in 2009, and has since spread his story at universities and rallies in Texas and beyond.

The obstacle that cannabis faces, as he sees it, is a gap in education. "It's very sad that people are afraid of what they don't understand, and that what they don't understand they restrict," he says.

He's considering a bid for the Texas state legislature in 2016, with cannabis at the top of his platform, and is pushing for increased access to cannabis for veterans.

"I didn't think I'd be thrust into the position I was thrust into," he says, "but if I could take it all back, I don't think I'd trade it in a second."

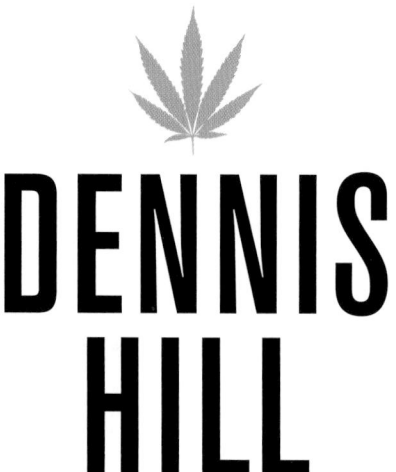

DENNIS HILL

Age 78 / **Stage III Adenocarcinoma** / Turnlock, California

"Did you know cannabis cures cancer?"

Dennis Hill was just a few days away from his first radiation appointment when a woman in one of his meditation classes posed this question to him. It was 2010, soon after he was diagnosed with Stage III Adenocarcinoma, a cancer of the glandular system that was concentrated in his prostate.

A former biochemist, Dennis had worked for 10 years in cancer research, including a period at M.D. Anderson Cancer Center in Houston, Texas, and yet was surprised by the woman's question. He answered something to the effect of, "No, I had no idea."

"During the years I was working in cancer research, from 1970 to 1980, all I knew about cannabis was that it was considered a toxic drug and you could be thrown in jail if you were caught with it," he says. "Nobody made that [medical] connection back then."

Intrigued, and already distrustful of radiation and chemotherapy, he immediately began researching medicinal cannabis use for cancer on the Internet. Although low in volume, the research he found was heartening enough that he cancelled his radiation appointment.

"In my work, I watched lots of people die from the conventional treatment," he says. "So when it was my turn, I had a choice, an educated choice, to go traditional and die from a treatment, or take a risk and go for the cannabis. Based on what I was able to learn and with my background I had confidence that this would work."

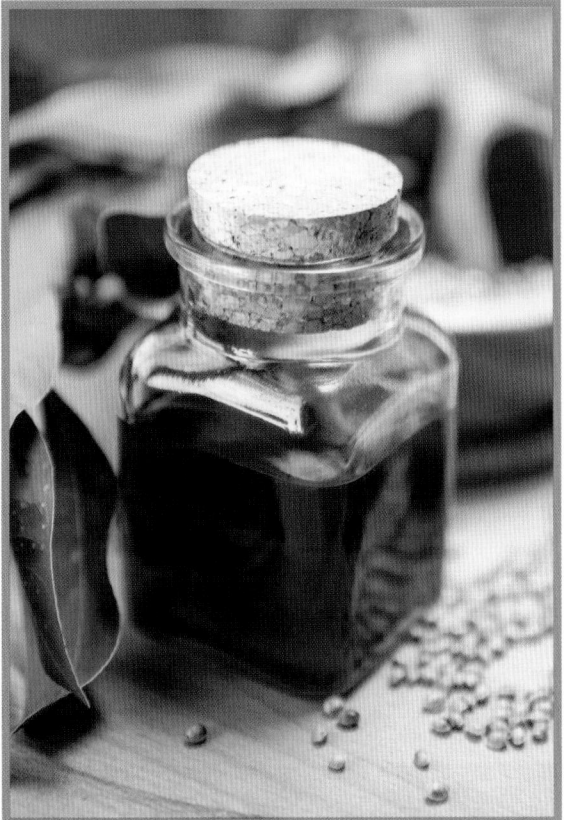

"THERE IS NO REASON TO BE AFRAID. IT'S GREAT MEDICINE."

Sure enough, he adds, it did. The primary tumor disappeared halfway through the six-month cannabis regimen on which he embarked, and remaining metastatic lesions soon followed suit. With no conventional medical intervention, he was clear of all cancer by the end of those six months.

It had been 30 years since Dennis used cannabis, but he still held a positive attitude about it. "I knew it was harmless," he says. "I had no fear of it, like a lot of people have. When I became convinced of the clinical benefits, then there were no barriers for me trying it."

At first, he ate a weak-potency butter made with cannabis plant trimmings. For the last leg, he used cannabis oil obtained from a medical marijuana co-op. Today, he uses a small amount of Rick Simpson Oil each night for maintenance. Although his internist was supportive of his choice of treatment, his urologist remained negative about it, even after his cancer disappeared. "He presumed it was a spontaneous remission," Dennis notes.

Dennis now frequently shares his story, often to others battling cancer and for whom he has two main pieces of advice: One, "Cannabis works—even if it's weak, you just take more. You don't have to wait for high-potency buds. Start with what you've got."

And two, the meditation teacher says it's important to have a good attitude about the plant if you want a successful outcome: "There is no reason to be afraid," he says. "It's great medicine."

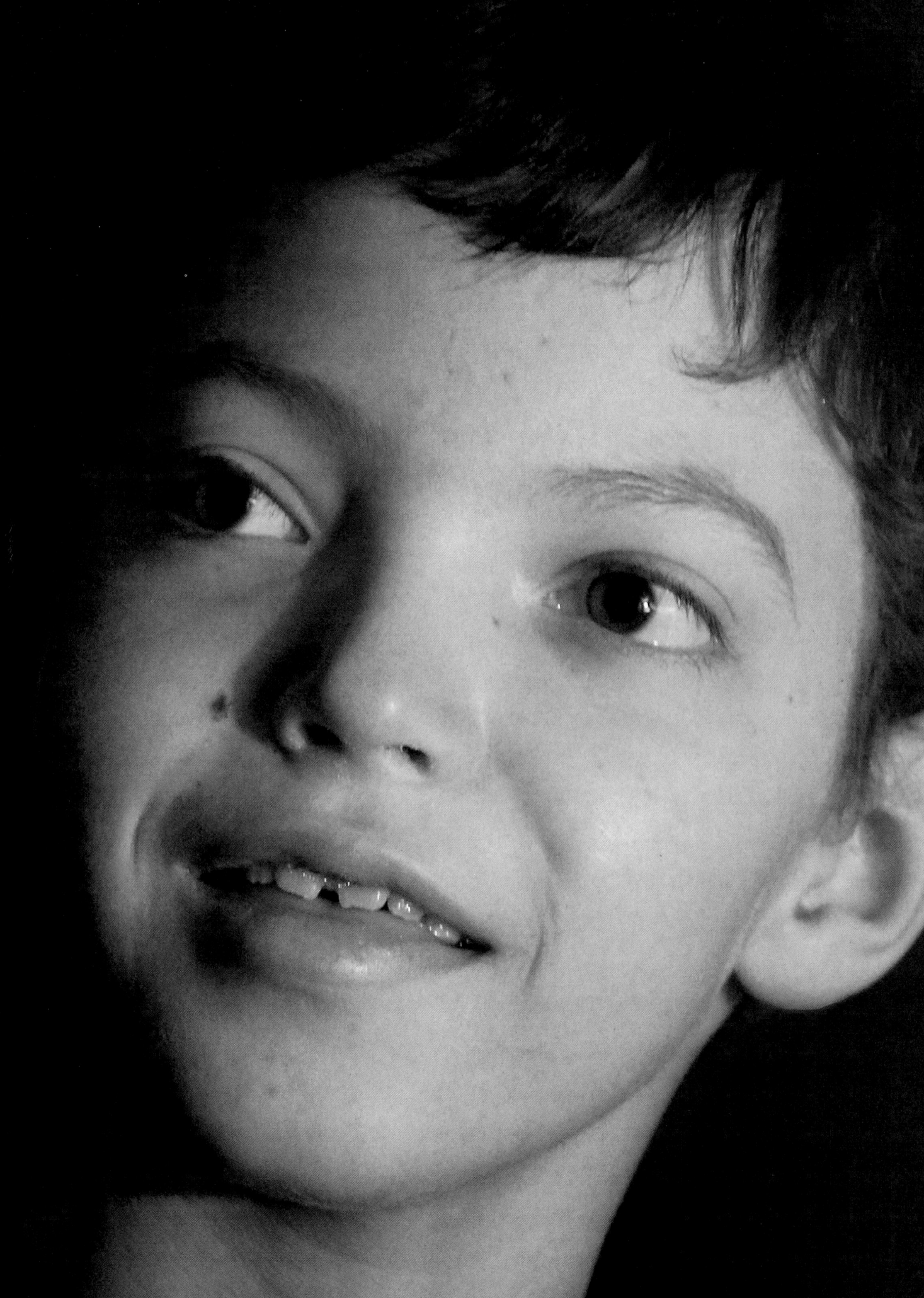

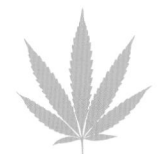

TYLER BROWN

Age 13 / Cerebral Palsy, Lennox-Gastaut syndrome / Monument, Colorado

"Quite frankly, ma'am, we aren't sure your son is going to make it." This wasn't news to Rita Brown when doctors at the Children's Hospital in Aurora, Colorado, told her in early 2012. She knew how fragile her son Tyler's life was at that point, and she knew they were running out of ways to help him.

When Tyler, now 13 years old, was checked into the hospital on Feb. 17 of that year, it seemed like it would be one of his routine visits. He'd contracted pneumonia after aspirating, or inhaling, food into his lungs, which happened so often that Tyler would spend about 10 days a month in the ICU during the late fall/ early winter respiratory season each year.

Born with cerebral palsy, Tyler was diagnosed at age 7 with a severe form of epilepsy called Lennox-Gastaut syndrome. At the time of this particular hospital visit, none of the medications or treatments tried thus far had quelled his 60 seizures a day. A seizure while he was eating could cause him to aspirate, and some medications he took increased aspirations.

"We were constantly in and out of the hospital," says Rita, who would stick by his side. "Month after month, every cold turned into pneumonia, every aspiration turned to pneumonia."

Soon after checking into the hospital in February 2012, Tyler entered status epileptics—a state in which the body is in constant seizure activity. "He was having a tonic clonic seizure every minute," Rita says. "Every minute it would start up again and stop." The mother-and-son duo were transferred to the Children's Hospital in Aurora, north of their home near Colorado Springs, where they stayed for three difficult months.

There, doctors attempted to control the seizures with IV-drip medications and a blood transfusion. Unsuccessful, they put him in a medically induced coma to allow his brain to rest. But the seizures started back up as soon as the coma was lifted a week later, and Tyler was put into coma No. 2.

Rita chokes up describing the experience. "It was the worst time of my life," she says.

Doctors presented Rita and her husband Jason with an eleventh-hour option: emergency brain surgery. Separating the two hemispheres of the brain could stop Tyler's seizures, but there was no guarantee.

"They said, 'We'll give you a moment to discuss it,'" Rita remembers. "My husband and I cried and we talked, and the surgeon came back and he said, 'If this were my child I'd do it.' We said 'OK.' They did the surgery the next day."

Back home near Colorado Springs, unbeknownst to the Browns, a little girl named Charlotte Figi was finding relief from her relentless, severe seizures with a low-THC, high-CBD cannabis oil. Charlotte would go on to become the poster child for pediatric medical cannabis and the eponym behind the now widely used oil Charlotte's Web. But cannabis wasn't on the Browns' radar—not yet.

"If we had only known. If we had only known," Rita repeats, tearfully. "But we didn't."

Brain surgery delivered the hoped-for results: Tyler's seizures ceased, and he was released from the hospital the day before Mother's Day, having endured heart and tracheotomy surgeries in addition to the brain operation.

"Unfortunately, he was completely wheelchair bound and had lost all form of communication," Rita says. "But he was alive."

Before his seizures started when he was 7, Tyler lived with cerebral palsy but was high-functioning.

"He was running up and down the stairs and playing and dancing," says Rita. "He was a pretty active, lively child. Very happy." Tyler had a small vocabulary—about 20 words—with which to

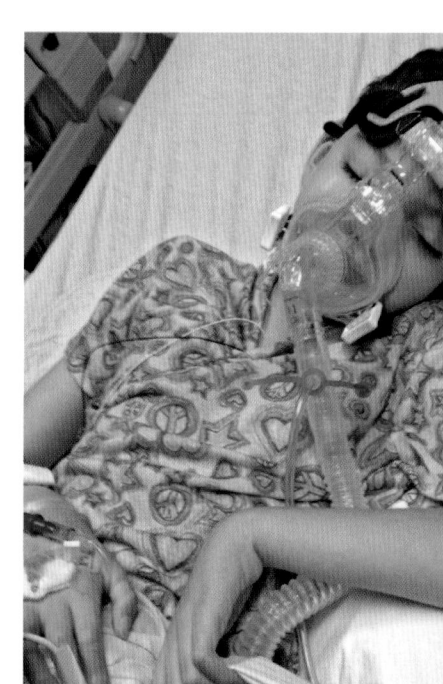

communicate and was in the process of potty training when he began suddenly dropping to the floor at random. At first, he'd get right back up and carry on, no problem. But soon he was falling a few times a week, and then every day. A series of 12 tried-and-failed medications followed his Lennox-Gastaut syndrome diagnosis, and all the while his seizures worsened—escalating to include every type of seizure, numbering 60 a day. The Ketogenic diet, a high-fat, low-carb way of eating designed to target hard-to-treat epilepsy, didn't help, nor did an implant—a vagus nerve stimulator (VNS)—that is supposed to send signals to the brain that interrupt seizures.

"Med after med after med we started losing his quality of life," Rita says. He fell so often, breaking his arms or getting concussions, that he was put in a wheelchair, and he lost what language he did have and fell into a cycle of chronic pneumonias.

Rita, who had quit her job at a children's psychiatric hospital after Tyler's first birthday, had the drill down. At the earliest sign of the sniffles, she packed her bags for the hospital, made a few meals, and called Tyler's school to excuse him for two weeks. She told her husband to alert his employer that he'd be working from home while caring for their other

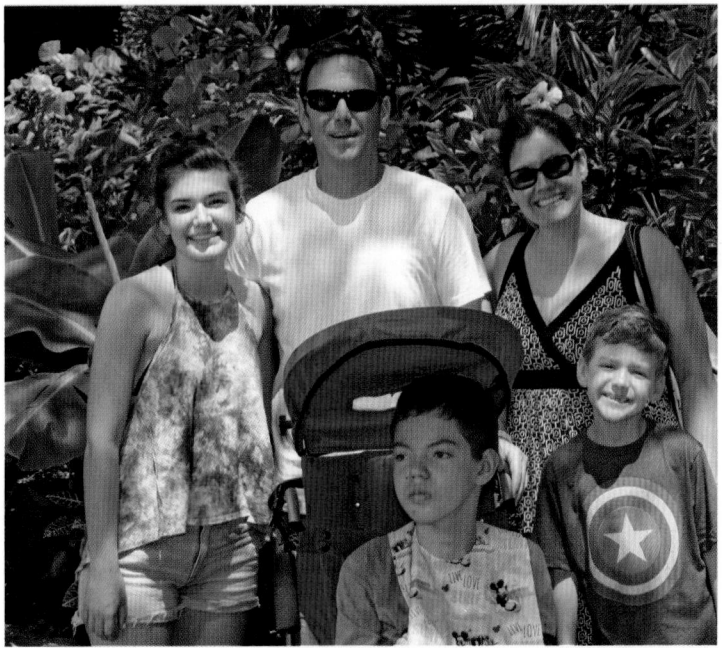

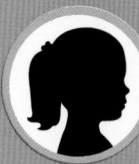 **CHARLOTTE'S WEB:** Charlotte's Web is a form of non-psychoactive cannabis oil used to treat seizures in children. The oil was named after Charlotte Figi, a 5-year-old girl who suffered from uncontrollable epileptic seizures. The only treatment that worked was a certain strain of CBD oil, which her mother said stopped 99.9 percent of the seizures. After Charlotte's story was featured in the 2013 CNN documentary *Weed*, other families started seeking the treatment, and Charlotte's Web is now sold commercially to help other epileptic children. The oil is also the inspiration behind the Charlotte's Web Medical Access Act, a bill under consideration by Congress that would remove the federal prohibition on marijuana strains that have little or no THC and therefore don't cause users to feel high. Source: Realm of Caring Foundation, Reset.me, Epilepsy Foundation of Colorado.

two children, a now-16-year-old sister named Alexandra and 7-year-old brother named Christian, while she stayed in the hospital with Tyler.

"Being in and out of the hospital every month is exhausting, and it's not just the hospital, it's the ICU—tubes down his throat and everything. It's physically and mentally draining," she says. "As a family, whenever Tyler would get sick, my other kids would start to panic: 'Mom how long will you be gone? When will we see you?' They have PTSD symptoms when Tyler starts getting sick."

Tyler was doing well enough after his brain surgery to return to his special education program that September. But one week later he was hospitalized with pneumonia, and it all began to unravel.

"The day he was about to be released, I saw him jump [a seizure activity], then I saw it again and I thought, 'Maybe this was a fluke,'" Rita says. "Then here we go again, once a week he's dropping [in a seizure]. And we can't do this again, because we've done everything—we've tried the medications, we've tried the diet, we've done the surgery, the VNS. We can't let the seizures start again. He had no quality of life with them."

It was back to the hospital in December, and again in January and in February. Meanwhile, his seizures crept upward in frequency, growing to as many as nine a day by the following summer. September arrived, and with it the earliest hint of respiratory season, and Tyler was once again hospitalized for pneumonia.

Just when the Browns thought they'd reached the end of their rope, they gained a few promising inches.

"Medicinal marijuana stops seizures, brings hope to a little Black Forest girl," read a headline in the Colorado Springs newspaper, *The Gazette*. The article detailed the astounding improvements Charlotte Figi experienced from using the oil that was eventually named after her.

"[My husband and I] opened up the paper, sat there and read it, and we were both in tears, saying, 'Oh my gosh. We have got to do this.'"

Luckily, the Browns lived just a short distance from the Colorado Springs organization responsible for Charlotte's Web: the Realm of Caring Foundation.

By October 2013, Tyler had his medical marijuana card and began his Charlotte's Web treatment. Today, Tyler still has up to nine seizures a day, but they are minor

"BEING IN AND OUT OF THE HOSPITAL EVERY MONTH IS EXHAUSTING, AND IT'S NOT JUST THE HOSPITAL, IT'S THE ICU—TUBES DOWN HIS THROAT AND EVERY-THING. IT'S PHYSICALLY AND MENTALLY DRAINING." —RITA BROWN, TYLER BROWN'S MOTHER

varieties and only seconds long. "He isn't having every type like he used to," says Rita. "We're not seeing 60 a day. I think the oil is keeping the seizures at bay."

The biggest benefit the oil brought Tyler was an unexpected one. "It was respiratory season when we started Charlotte's Web," Rita explains. "We'd just gotten out of the hospital in September with pneumonia. In October, we started Charlotte's Web and a week later he got a cold and I thought, 'Here we go.' I started packing my bags. And I waited ... Nothing. The next morning he still had his cold, and I kept him home from school, my bags still packed, and I called my husband and told him to work from home for the week. But day two goes by and he was fine, it was just a cold. Day three, his cold was gone. I was floored."

This was unheard of in the Brown family. Another uneventful cold followed in November, and then a cold with an accompanying fever in December—a sure-fire pneumonia, the parents thought. But the fever subsided and Tyler was on the mend. Soon, respiratory season had passed without a single visit to the hospital.

He hasn't set foot in a hospital since.

Tyler is back in school now, where another kid can sneeze or cough on him without need for panic. He no longer needs to be hooked up to oxygen at night, as he did before Charlotte's Web, and he has stopped seeing his pulmonary doctor and cardiologist. In a major boon to his

well-being, Rita has been able to wean him off of other medications.

"He was on four meds and he couldn't hold his head up, he drooled. His quality of life was nonexistent on those medications. He was drugged up and comatose, really," she says. Now she says he's alert and interactive. Happy, even.

"The Tyler I have now, he's still wheelchair bound, but I see his life coming back," she says. "He's so much more interactive and I think he's happier. I can see it in his eyes. He's definitely in a better place. We still have two medications to go, and I can't wait to see where we are without those, because they are still fogging his brain. I have hope that someday he'll walk and talk again. There's still hope."

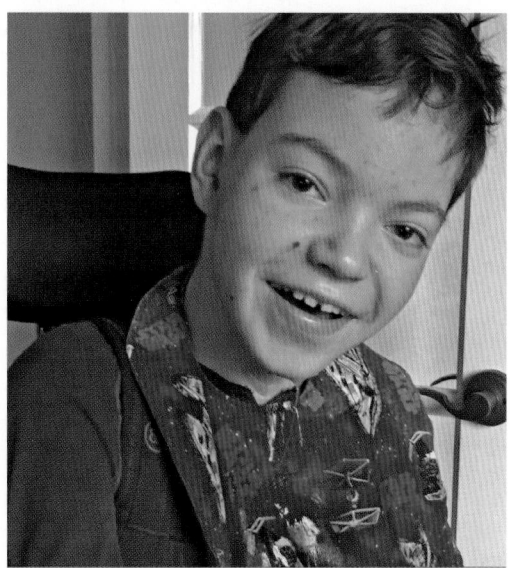

"I SEE HIS LIFE COMING BACK. HE'S SO MUCH MORE INTERAC-TIVE AND I THINK HE'S HAPPIER. I CAN SEE IT IN HIS EYES."
—RITA BROWN

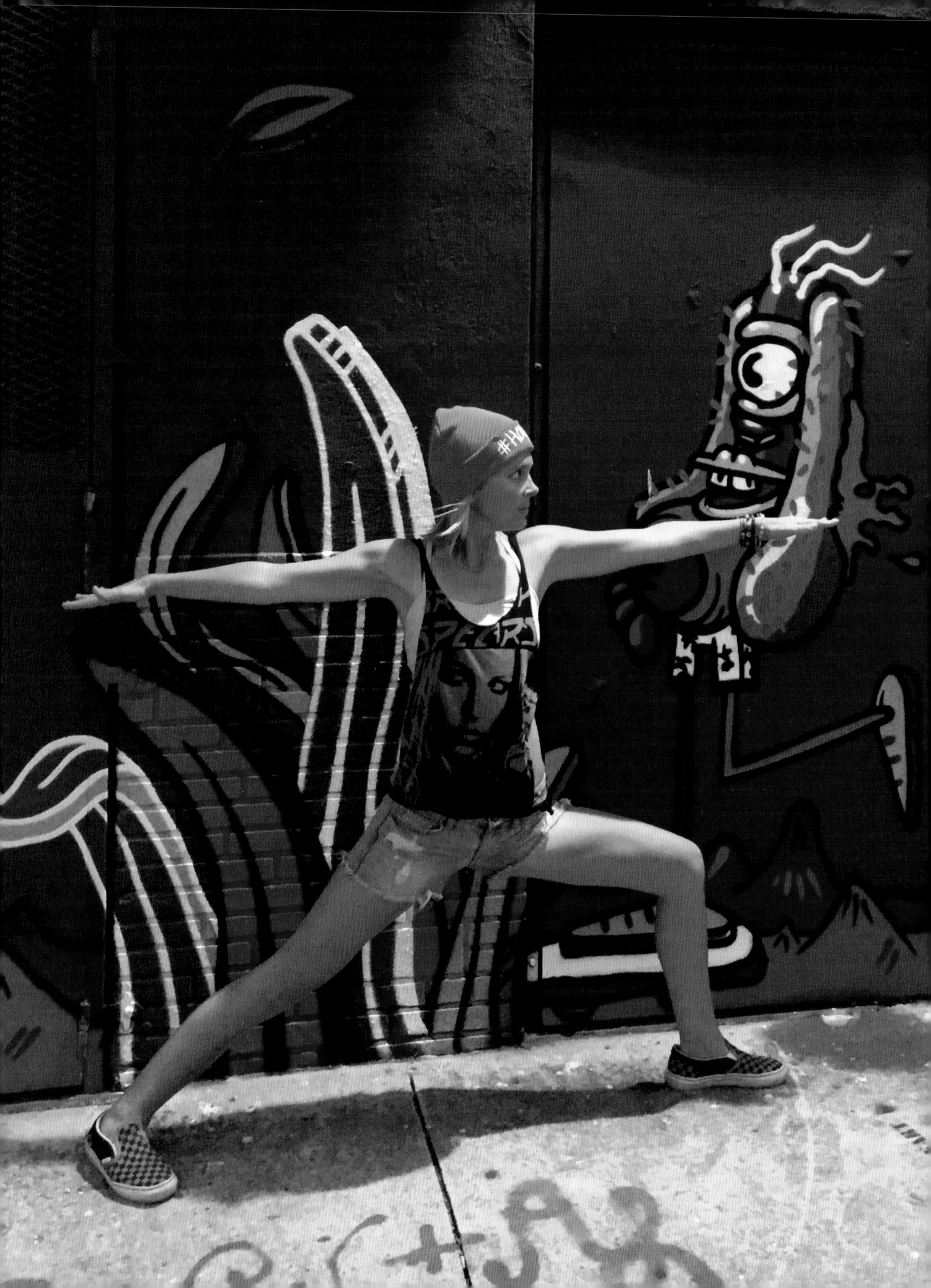

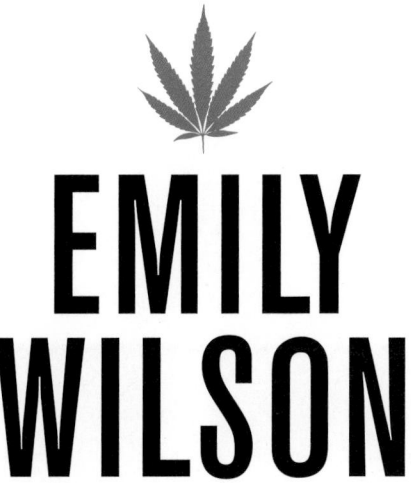

EMILY WILSON

Age 36 / **Pectus Excavatum** / Fort Lauderdale, Florida

All her life, Emily Wilson's doctors assured her that her concave chest was solely a cosmetic problem.

The 36-year-old has had pectus excavatum—a condition in which a person's breastbone is sunken into his or her chest—as long as she can remember. But it was as a teenager that it began causing her problems.

"I remember I was about 16 and I was wearing a swimsuit," Emily recalls. "My sister said 'What happened to you?' I never knew anything was wrong."

Clothes didn't fit right, and the undesirable reality of being different than other teens weighed heavily on her. Physical exertion became difficult, and she was forced to sit and watch as her friends and peers did activities she couldn't.

Years later, she learned this was because the caved chest was putting pressure on her heart, restricting the flow of oxygen. But until then, her complaints to doctors about shortness of breath, back pain and severe migraines were met with a litany of prescriptions—seven pills taken daily, including a 12-year run of Prozac to curb the despair she felt, and a handful that were used as needed.

"Anything that can go wrong if your heart doesn't pump right went wrong," she says. "Through all the complaining they just kept medicating me."

Two major surgeries in 2009—a hysterectomy aimed at alleviating endometriosis, and the removal of a non-cancerous brain tumor—didn't help with her chronic problems. She could barely make it up a flight of stairs.

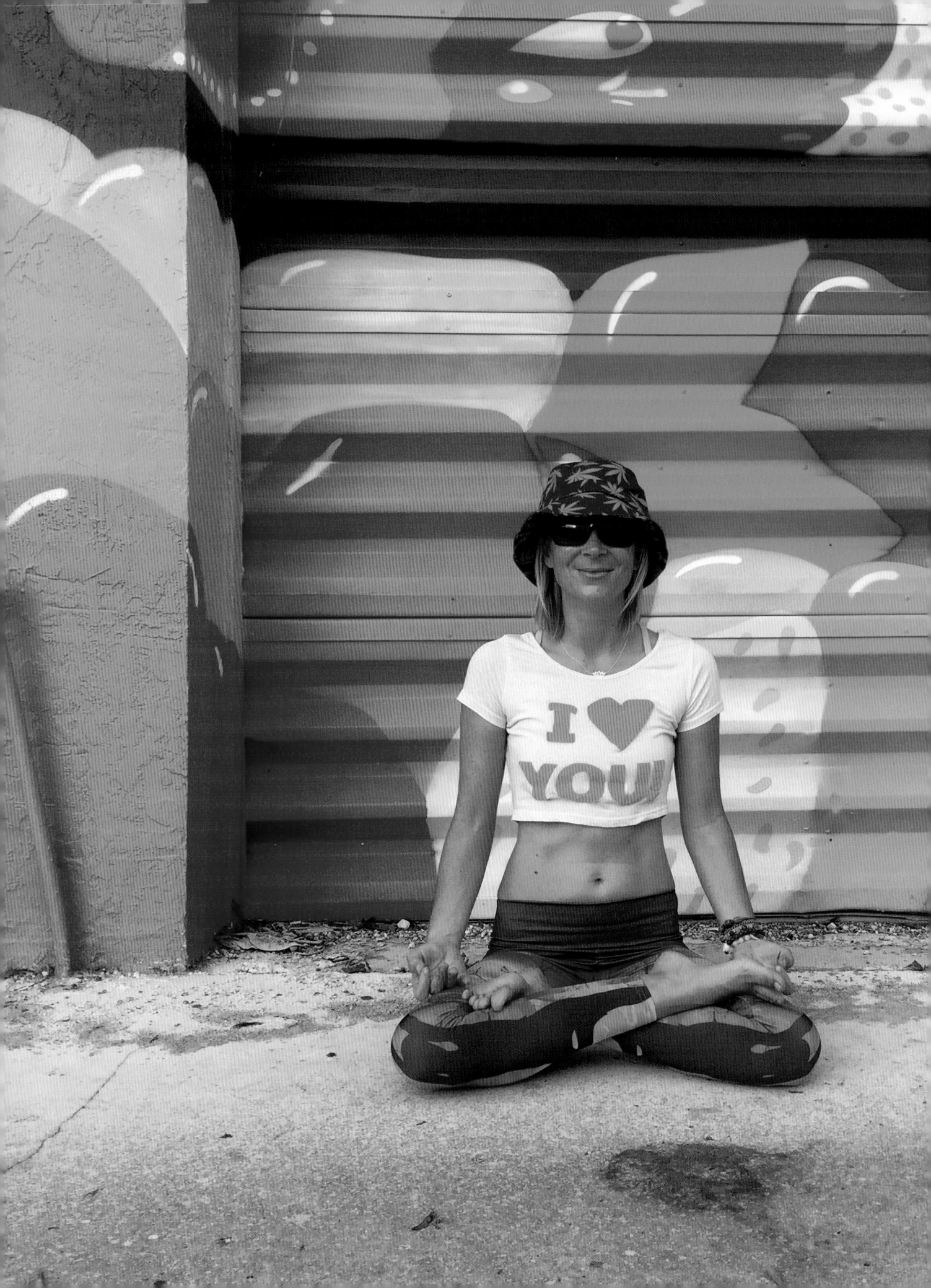

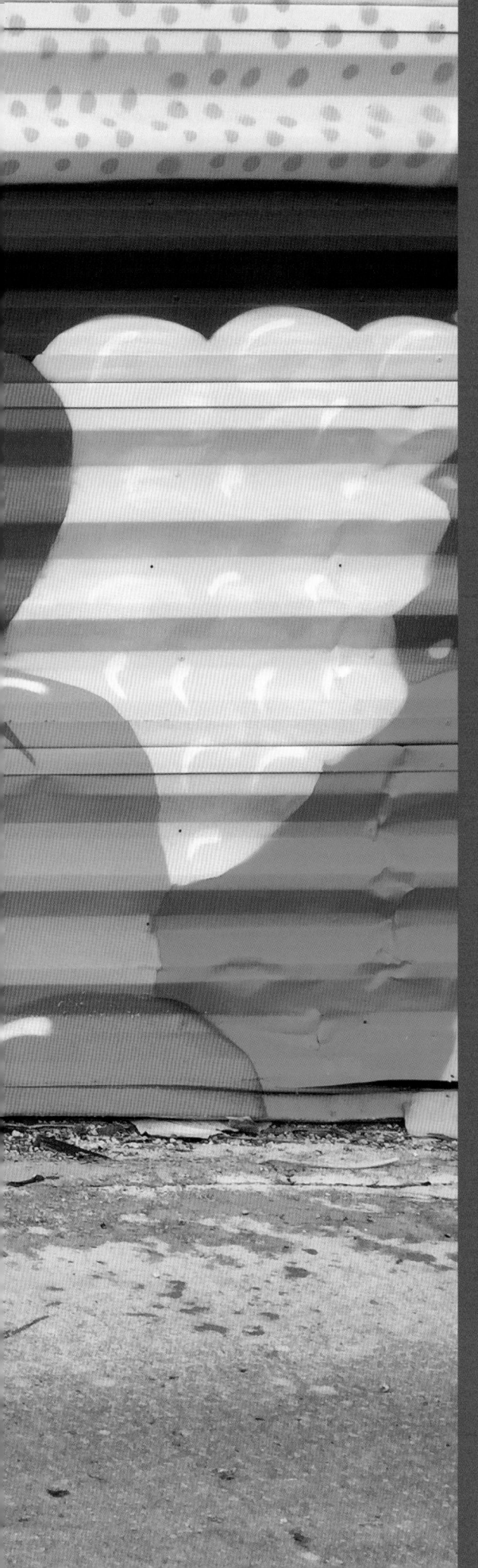

"WAKING UP IS PAINFUL. YOU REALIZE, 'MAN, I WAS LIED TO [ABOUT CANNABIS BEING BAD].' THAT REALIZATION WAS ROUGH—CONSIDERING ALL THOSE YEARS ON ALL THAT MEDICINE, AND ALL THE DAMAGE IT DID TO ME PHYSICALLY, EMOTIONALLY AND MENTALLY."

Finally, at age 33, a doctor agreed to do an MRI. It revealed a bowling-pin shaped heart, pinched small at one end and bulging at the other, and lungs the size of a 7-year-old's. She was diagnosed with pectus excavatum and, a few months later in January 2013, underwent the first of two surgeries to address it. Surgeons broke her sternum, removed six ribs, and placed a bar across her chest to be worn until the ribs grew back. After the second surgery in June of that year, she was still miserable.

"I sat in my house—I couldn't be away from my heating pad," she says. "It hurt to stand. The only thing that felt decent was [laying] on my back in my bed on my heating pad. When you're in pain, you're irritable. I was angry a lot."

Emily looked at her life and the unbearable discomfort she faced each day and decided to do whatever she could to "make my body work better." She read up on healthy living, saw documentaries about food, and started eating better. She watched yoga videos and hoped that someday she could do it herself. Medical marijuana cropped up in her research, spurring her to try smoking

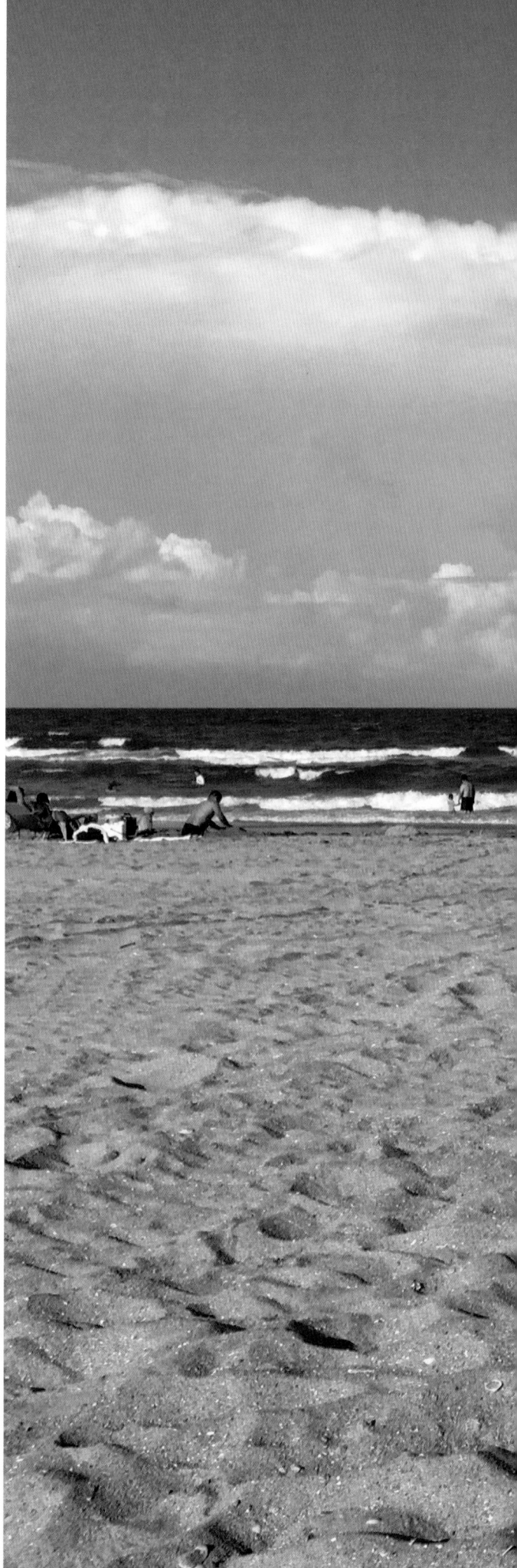

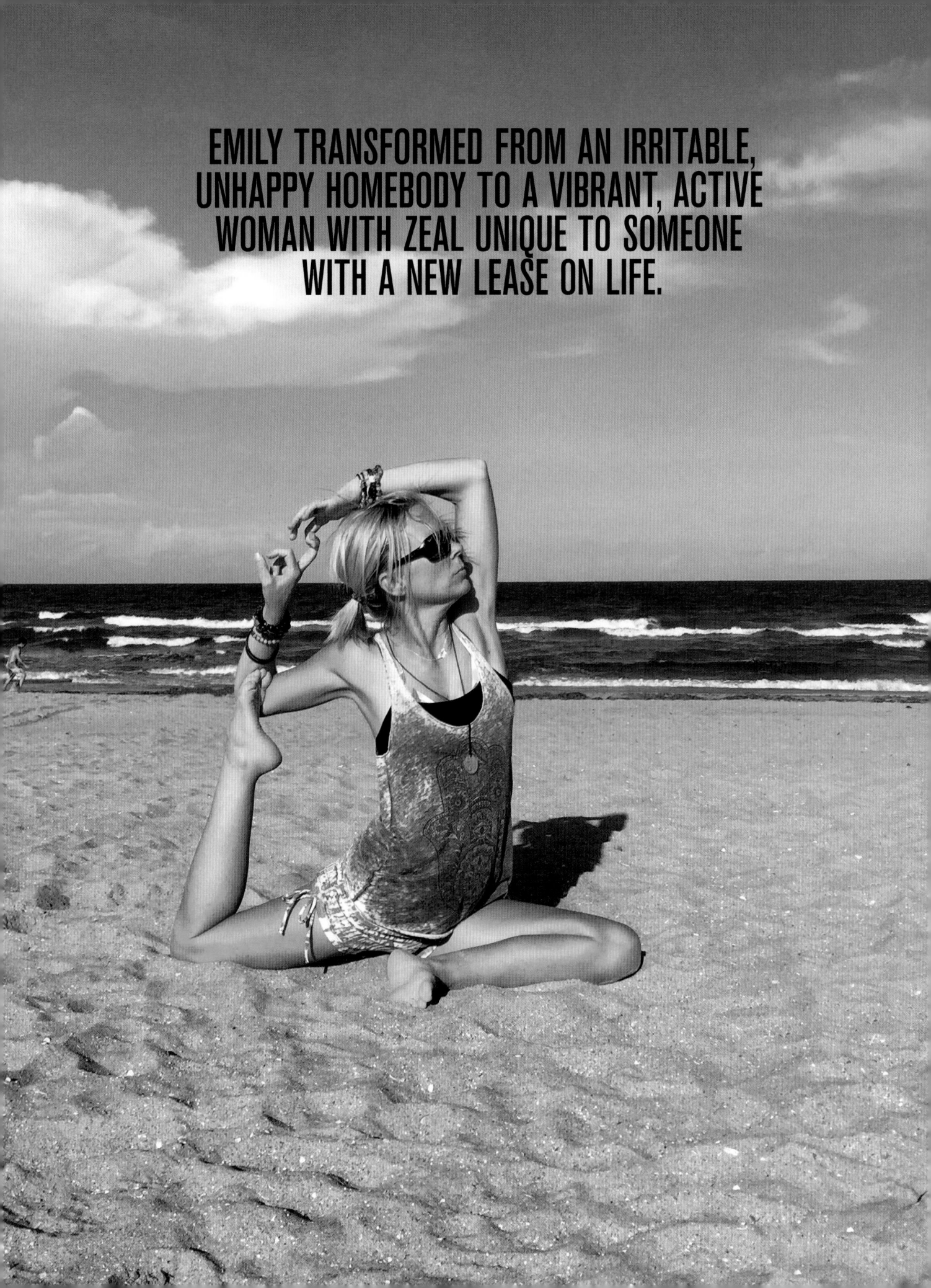

EMILY TRANSFORMED FROM AN IRRITABLE, UNHAPPY HOMEBODY TO A VIBRANT, ACTIVE WOMAN WITH ZEAL UNIQUE TO SOMEONE WITH A NEW LEASE ON LIFE.

it for the first time in many years. While it was pleasant, she didn't experience the sort of results she had read about online.

"I started looking into other ways to take it because two hits a night wasn't going to fix missing ribs," says Emily, who managed to find some Rick Simpson Oil, which aided with the excruciating pain of growing new ribs.

One night soon after beginning to ingest the cannabis oil, Emily forgot to take Prozac, which had been part of her daily routine for more than a decade. Five days later she realized she still hadn't taken it. After six weeks, she was off of all other medications, "just because I didn't need them," she says matter-of-factly. To her surprise, she experienced no withdrawals or side effects from cutting off pharmaceuticals that had been pumping through her body for years.

The life ruled by pain and lived in anger faded away. Emily transformed from an irritable, unhappy homebody to a vibrant, active woman with zeal unique to someone with a new lease on life.

She tells her story in hurried excitement, as if she can't get the happy news out fast enough. Her focus now is on yoga—the embodiment of just how far she's come. Something she had always wished she could do became a reality, and it helped her health even more by opening up her chest. Yoga captured her heart so much that she became instructor, and while there are still some poses her body can't quite do, like a full back bend, she's confident she will master them eventually. She started a company with two friends called The Traveling Yoginis, and is traversing the country in a decked-out camper van, teaching yoga to sick and injured people for free along the way.

What does she hope others can learn from her experience? "That you don't have to live like I was living," she says. "Waking up is painful. You realize, 'Man, I was lied to [about cannabis].' That realization was rough—considering all those years on all that medicine, and all the damage it did to me physically, emotionally and mentally, it made me mad in the beginning. Like, 'I wasted my whole life.' Now I'm feeling like I'm only 36. I'm young, I'm healthy. I have a lot of years left to help a lot of people. Now that I feel good, it's a gift I don't want to waste."

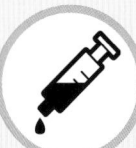

RICK SIMPSON OIL: In 2003, Rick Simpson discovered that hemp oil was an effective cure for his basil cell carcinoma skin cancer. Since then he has spread the word to encourage others to benefit from the medicine as he has. Simpson starred in the documentary *Run From the Cure*, and provides free instructions on how to create the oil on his website PhoenixTears.ca. Simpson considers his oil a preventative medicine that promotes full body healing, and can help ward off diseases like diabetes, cancer and multiple sclerosis (MS) before they start. *Source: PhoenixTears.ca.*

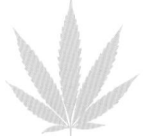

I.L.

Age 38 / **PTSD** / Gilbert, Arizona

Even though I.L. obtains medical cannabis legally as a card-carrying patient in Arizona, "there's still a stigma out there," she says. And for this reason, she has asked that only her initials be used to identify her.

"I'm still very private about it," says I.L., who served in the U.S. Navy from 1996 to 2005. "How you choose to medicate is a very personal thing. It's not so much that I feel like I'm doing something wrong, it's everyone else's feelings about it. Those attitudes are based on decades of misinformation."

Consequently, she hasn't revealed her cannabis use to most of her family or friends, and keeps it from those at the large tech company where she works as a technician. She does, however, spend much of her time sharing information and resources about cannabis with fellow veterans (albeit anonymously) through the Veterans Cannabis Collective, a vol-

unteer-run online community she co-founded in December 2014. She wants to spread the word that cannabis can be a healing modality for veterans, whether they suffer from PTSD, as she does, or other ailments.

As is the case for most veterans, the fighting didn't end when I.L. returned to civilian life. It was simply the start of a second act—a war of personal battles.

Enlisting in the Navy had been a no-brainer for I.L.—she was following in a family tradition that included two brothers, her father and her grandfather—and, for much of her nine-year term, she believed she would make a career of it. That path was unfolding before her, as she received promotions and climbed higher on the ladder. By Sept. 11, 2001, she was a leading petty officer with up to 15 people reporting to her.

"I remember that day like it was yesterday," she says. Upon hearing that planes had hit the World Trade Center, the mood immediately switched on the aircraft carrier she was on. Already at sea, the ship was rerouted for New York. "It was, 'OK, we're at war,'" she says. The vessel was turned around before reaching New York (enough other ships arrived sooner), but I.L. and her shipmates were soon deployed to the Persian Gulf, for the first of two times, in January 2002, where I.L. worked on weapon systems.

"We were dropping bombs day and night," I.L. remembers. "Literally, planes were flying off the carrier nonstop, and they were loaded. They were ready to go."

Tensions were high for the duration of the experience, and I.L. ran on vigilant, detached autopilot. "For me, in a leadership position, my personal feelings had to be set aside," she says. "There was no time for me to think or feel. People are looking to me to see how I respond."

The actual events of being at war, and the distress of living under those conditions for a sustained period of time, planted the seeds for the severe anxiety and PTSD that sprouted once I.L. returned home. But there was another factor at work in creating her discontent, and it ultimately led her to change her mind about a career in the Navy.

"The most painful thing for me was realizing, 'Wait a minute, maybe we're not right,'" she says. "I saw it: dropping bombs, launching aircraft, and I thought, 'There is no way we aren't harming and killing innocent people.' It was this weird shift. It got really uncomfortable for me."

It was because of this epiphany that she left the Navy in 2005, settling in Arizona, where she began the long journey of recovering from the experience.

"A lot of the anxiety is [from] the hyper vigilance. You're always on edge, always ready for the worst," she says. "When I got out, it took me years to calm down." After a long game of prescription drug whack-a-mole, in which one side effect pops up and another drug is thrown into the mix to shove it back down, she had a change of heart.

"I thought there is just something wrong when I can get buckets filled and no one questions that," she says. She was undergoing a lifestyle shift toward organic food, meditation and other natural interests, and taking pharmaceuticals no longer fit in.

Today, she medicates with cannabis— mostly edibles, or food items made with marijuana or marijuana oils—and is tapering off her other prescriptions.

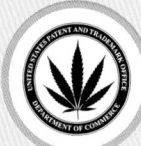

PATENTS: There are about 1,660 patents in the United States related to cannabis, according to Google Patent Search. The U.S. Department of Health and Human Services was granted a patent in 2003 for "Cannabinoids as antioxidants and neuroprotectants," which acknowledges their utility against stroke, Alzheimer's disease, Parkinson's disease and dementia, according to the U.S. Patent and Trademark Office.

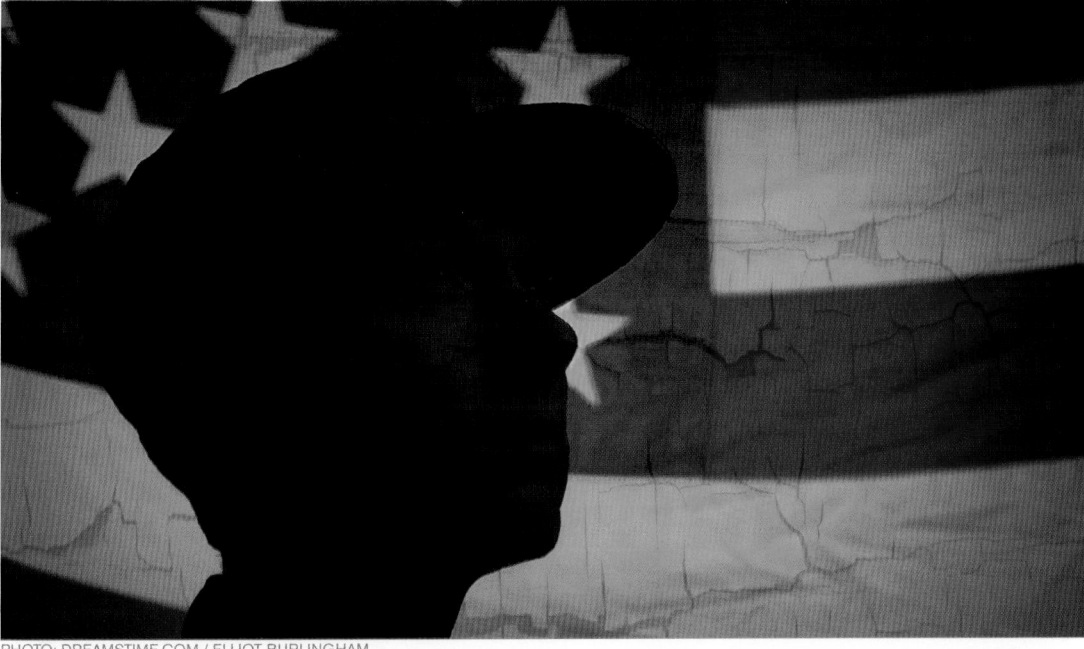

PHOTO: DREAMSTIME.COM / ELLIOT BURLINGHAM

"VETERANS NEED A LIFELINE. THEY NEED TO KNOW THERE ARE OTHER OPTIONS. THEY NEED TO KNOW IT'S OK—THAT THERE IS HOPE OUT THERE."

"The best way I can describe [cannabis] for me is that it restores a sense of balance and peace," she says.

Through her recent outreach, I.L. has found that other veterans are just as fed up with the prescription deluge as she was. "I found a sense of camaraderie and, really, a sense of the desperation within the veteran community. We are tired of being prescribed pills all the time," she says. "From day one in boot camp, they prescribe 800mg Tylenol. You can get anything really. They have no qualms about prescribing these medications and, in my opinion, creating addictions."

Her group, the Veterans Cannabis Collective, promotes cannabis as one component of a healing lifestyle that also includes whole, natural foods, meditation, and healthy habits.

"Quite frankly, it's terrifying for me to talk about [my cannabis use]," she says. "I'm really [talking about it] for my veteran community. Veterans need a lifeline. They need to know there are other options. They need to know it's OK—that there is hope out there."

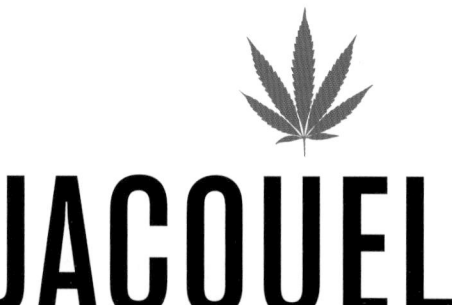

JACQUELINE PATTERSON

Age 36 / **Cerebral Palsy, Chronic Pain** / Marin County, California

For the estimated 760,000 Americans with cerebral palsy, the disability, which includes a number of neurological disorders, can have various implications on movement, mobility and muscle coordination.

For 36-year-old Jacqueline Patterson, it manifests as muscle spasms that cause her to speak with a severe stutter and generally makes the right side of her body hard to use. She also wrestles with chronic neck and back pain resulting from a neck injury in 1999. Without medication, she's too tense and in too much pain to lead a normal life.

"It makes daily activities like cleaning, taking care of the kids and otherwise having a life way more difficult," says the mother of four, three of whom live with her in Marin County, California. Conventional prescription medications may ease the pain, but they also create new problems: "On pharmaceuticals, I can't move because I'm all doped up," she says.

She's found that cannabis is powerfully effective for pain relief and reducing muscle spasticity and doesn't carry the same inhibitive side effects. As it relaxes those rigid muscles on her right side, she's able to do otherwise unmanageable tasks like brush and style her own hair, and—most importantly—she can express herself with greater fluency. "Without using cannabis, the muscles that I speak with are very spastic, so it makes it really hard to communicate with people, especially people who have never experienced a stutter before," she says.

She prefers using topical cannabis products, which alleviate tension when

"IT'S NOT RIGHT TO MAKE PATIENTS MOVE ACROSS THE COUNTRY."

rubbed on her muscles. One dose of the sticky resin-like cannabis concentrate provides the pain relief and muscle relaxation equivalent to five joints over four hours, she says.

Jacqueline's history of medicating with cannabis began when she was a teenager and has been paved with many obstacles and sacrifices since. As a youth, no one except the friends she smoked marijuana with believed her that it made such a drastic difference in her condition. When the butt end of a joint was discovered in her backpack, Jacqueline was institutionalized in a juvenile mental health facility.

Years later, she made the difficult decision to uproot her life and move with her four children from their home in Kansas City, Missouri, to California so she could medicate legally. But when Jacqueline was served with child custody paperwork for her son Jade, she decided to stay in the Midwest and move closer to his father in Iowa. There, she was arrested for possession and, later, visited by Child Protective Services and told she should relocate to a cannabis-friendly state if she wished to continue using it. "That's what it took to drag me out here," says Jacqueline, who made the move in January 2007.

"I was perfectly content to stay and work it out until it was legal there, too."

In California, she struggled to find affordable housing and ran into some administrative problems for low-income housing vouchers that led to a 10-month period of homelessness, during which time Jade was sent to live with his father in Iowa, where he has lived since.

"There are times when I wonder if it's really worth it," she says, "and I think about packing it all up and moving to Iowa and just fighting for safe access and not having safe access, myself, until it gets passed there."

Having one's family torn apart is a possible consequence of being a medical marijuana refugee. The burden of moving, in general, is already disproportionately heftier for people with disabilities and illnesses. Not only does the stress and effort of moving add to already difficult lives, it means being cut off from existing support systems and resources, like family, friends, medical care, and in-home support. Not to mention that moving is an expensive, sizable obstacle for those who are too sick or disabled to work.

Simply put, Jacqueline says, "It's not right to make patients move across the country."

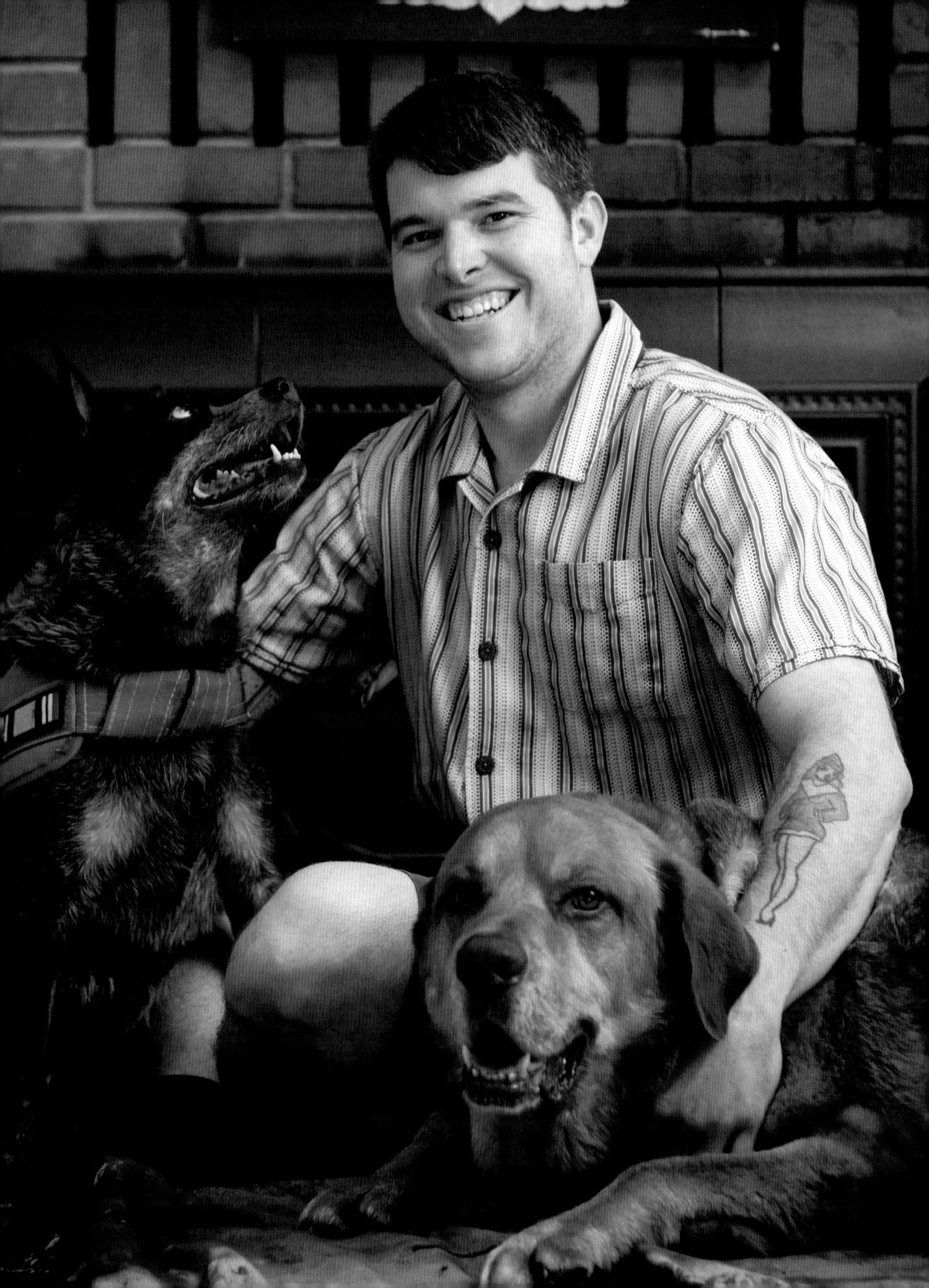

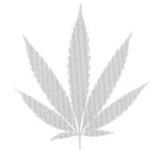

JAKE SCALLAN

Age 28 / **PTSD** / Bonny Doon, California

Picture a terrorist act as depicted on the evening news—the scattered chaos, the confusing eruption of sudden violence. That's the kind of action Jake Scallan saw all the time during his service in Iraq from June to December 2009.

As part of the United States Air Force security forces, the Californian kept guard at the north entrance of the base where he was stationed. Often, he was posted up in a security tower with a 50-caliber sniper rifle, scanning the boundaries for trouble and looking after the troops manning the perimeter. Sometimes he was part of that patrol himself, circling the base with an M2 machine gun.

For the modern combat soldier, every moment is lived in the trenches and every place they step is a potential bat-

tlefield. There's no march to the fight; no war cry to signal when it's time. Just an unpredictable succession of random attacks. As such, Jake lived in high alert, hyper aware of his surroundings and the moment-to-moment possibility of violence. "It would always be over just as fast as it started," he says.

The sum of it all—of being shot at with rifle fire while on patrol and in the guard tower, of seeing and hearing mortar and rocket explosions, of existing in a permanent state of heightened adrenaline and alertness—battered his mind and spirit.

When his deployment ended in December 2009, Jake was placed at a base in Oklahoma, a state with such unique climate conditions that it has a greater frequency of severe weather than nearly any

"I'VE REALLY SEEN THE WHOLE TRANSFORMATION, THE 180 [DEGREE CHANGE]. IT'S PHENOMENAL."

—EFFIE COBARRUBIA

other place on the planet. Thunderstorms, in particular, are a hallmark of Oklahoma skies, and the persistent soundtrack of booming thunder and cracks of lightning revealed Jake's PTSD right away.

"I remember a lot of sleepless nights because of thunderstorms," he says, sitting beside his fiancée, Effie Cobarrubia, at an expansive wooden table on the outdoor patio of a Santa Cruz, California, coffeehouse, with a wall of exposed brick behind them. Under the table at their feet is Bandit, a one-eyed, 4-year-old Blue Heeler that Jake adopted soon after moving off the Oklahoma base.

Doctors at the base diagnosed Jake with PTSD, along with depression and anxiety, and set him on a course of prescriptions and therapies. Some of it was helpful, particularly the prolonged-exposure therapy—a method based on facing one's fears head on. For Jake, this involved addressing his fear of hospitals, a result of an experience he had in Iraq, when he had been admitted to a hospital for pneumonia. A soldier who had been hit in the face by an IED, or improvised explosive device, was rushed into the room. Jake watched in horror as he died.

"That really messed with me," he says. "I went through [prolonged exposure] just to be able to go into hospitals again. It was rough stuff but it was really positive."

Zoloft, Klonopin and Seroquel, to name just a few of the prescriptions he was given, weren't as encouraging. He suspects that doctors loaded him up on these in part to subdue his increasingly defiant, angsty attitude. "I was real gruff and mean and rough around the edges to people who didn't go through a similar experience as me," he says.

Before enlisting, Jake described himself as gregarious, outgoing, even goofy. But that stressful, first-and-only six-month deployment was enough to rewire him to be short-tempered, tense and remote. "A lot of guys say this—it's something that, once it's turned on, it can't be turned off," he says.

Jake was released from the base and lived nearby while the military determined when he would be fit for duty.

Bandit, while not an official service dog, was Jake's loyal companion and protector. "There have been a lot of hard nights this dog has gotten me through," he says, reaching a tattooed arm under the table to ruffle Bandit's brown-and-gray fur, which is partially covered by a harness vest with "Scallan," his last name, emblazoned across the side. After a year and a half in limbo, the military medically retired Jake for PTSD in 2011.

Eager to leave that chapter in the dust, he packed up his car, Bandit in tow, and headed for his hometown of Fremont, California, where he moved in with his father. Life wasn't any cheerier in the Golden State, however—at least not at first.

New doctors looked at what he had been prescribed at the military base and replicated the list. One of Jake's best friends, a civilian, confronted him about how diminished he was when he was taking these drugs. "He said, 'Sometimes when you're on your meds, I can't understand what you're talking about,'" Jake remembers. The friend suggested Jake try smoking cannabis, which he did.

"Right away, it felt like I could breathe and take a step back," Jake says. "When I'm not medicating with cannabis, she can

attest to it"—he gestures at Effie, who nods in agreement—"I'm very snappy."

He obtained a medical marijuana license and became serious about finding out which strains and intake methods worked best for him. Coincidentally, a job search resulted in taking a security position at a medical marijuana collective in San Jose.

Around this time, however, his mental health issues reached a new low. Overworked, stressed, and grappling with problems in his personal life, Jake and Effie decided in the fall of 2013 that he should check into a VA psych ward for suicide watch.

"It was truly a *One Flew Over the Cuckoo's Nest* situation," Jake says. Between the stark white surroundings, cold floors, bright lights, strong-armed push of psychiatric meds, and a zero-tolerance attitude toward cannabis, Jake saw in clear terms that veterans weren't being given tools and space for actual healing. One upshot of his 10-day stint was that he felt the benefits of connecting with other veterans, even those whose experiences were different than

VETERANS & CANNABIS: Soldiers returning from Iraq, Afghanistan and other combat zones often suffer from ailments that cannabis can help treat, like pain, anxiety and post-traumatic stress disorder. However, doctors who work in the Veterans Administration system are barred by federal law from recommending marijuana to their patients. As a result, veterans who rely on the VA system for their healthcare have no way to legally access a medicine that can help them control their symptoms. Some veterans groups are advocating to change the rule, and Congress is currently considering a bill that would allow VA doctors to recommend medical marijuana to patients in states where it is legal. *Sources: Veterans for Medical Cannabis Access, Drug Policy Alliance.*

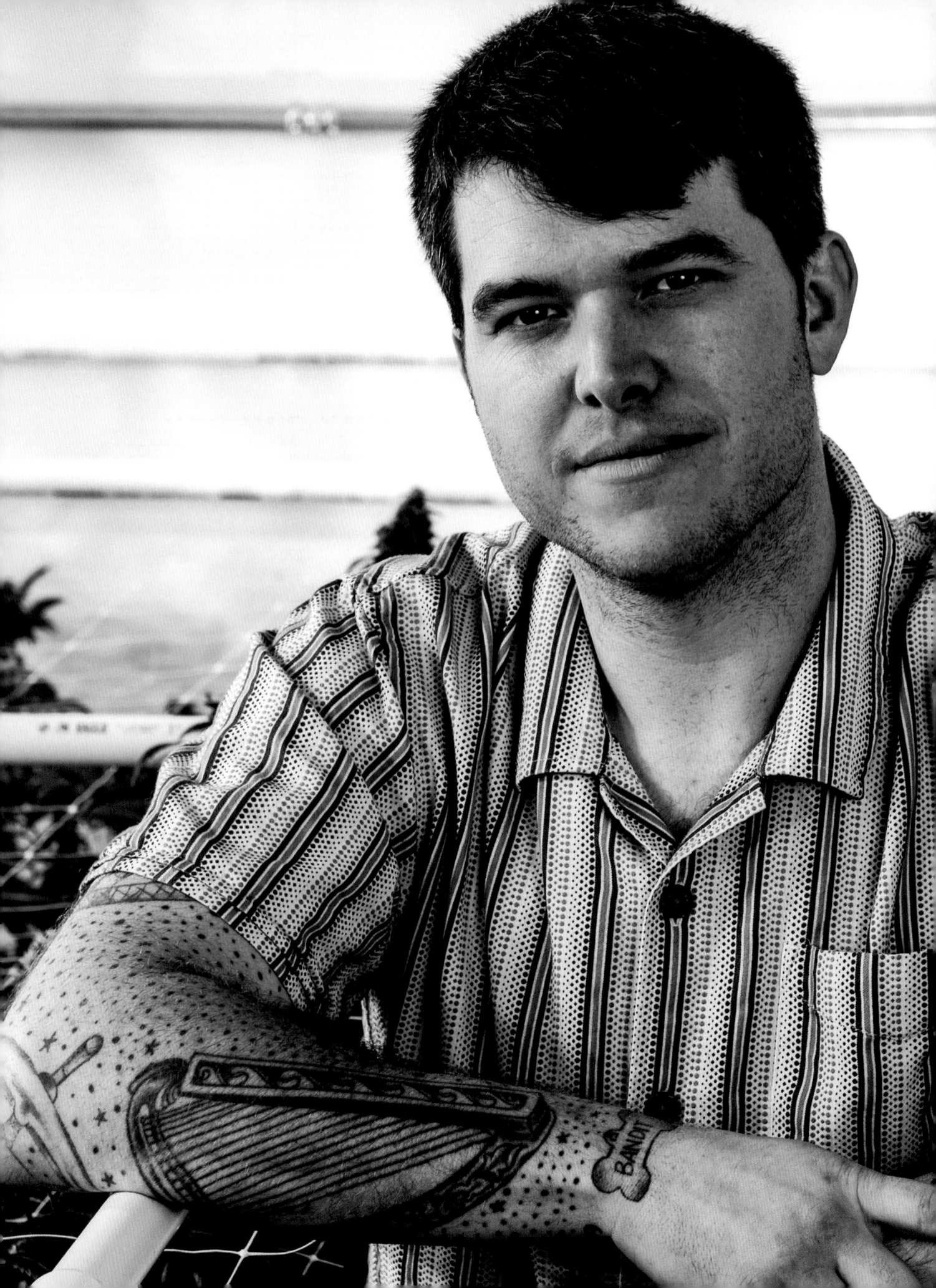

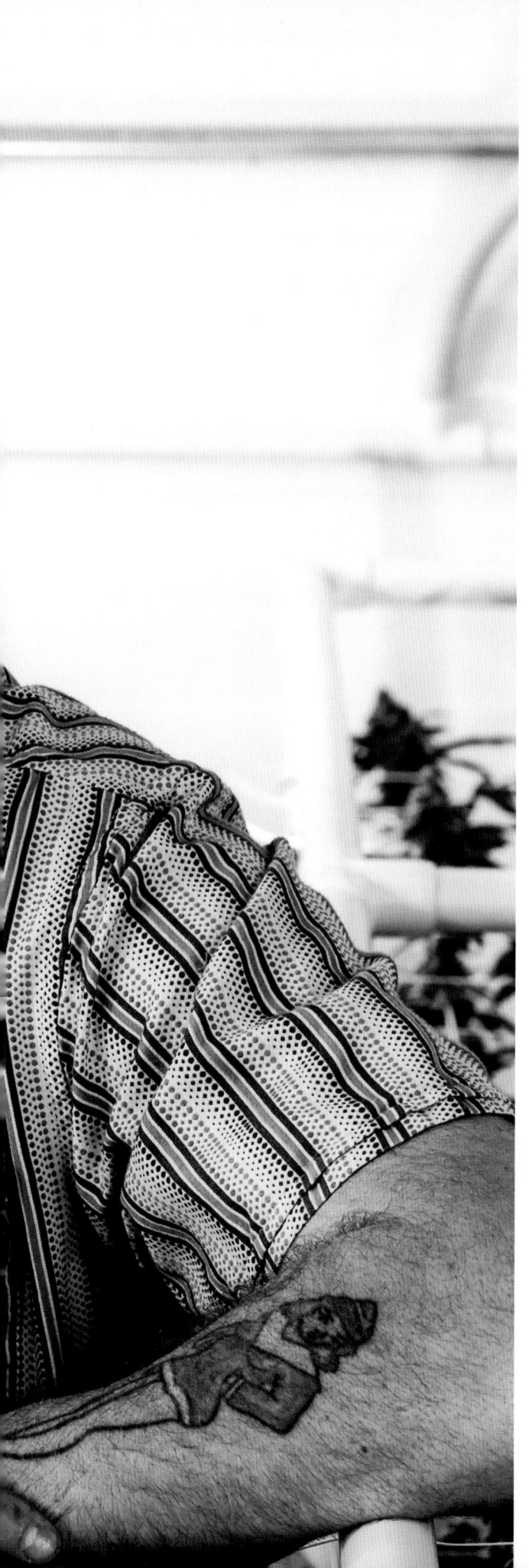

"[PTSD] IS STILL VERY MUCH A PART OF MY LIFE. THERE ARE GOOD DAYS AND BAD DAYS. CANNABIS LETS ME HANDLE THE TRIGGERS, ALLOWS ME TO ACKNOWLEDGE THEM."

his own. "It allowed me to understand another veteran's struggle, even if it isn't combat related," he says.

The day of his release, Jake happened to meet one of his heroes, Gulf War veteran and musician Mike McColgan. Jake points down to his shirt, a black graphic tee for the band Street Dogs, which McColgan fronts (he was also the original lead signer of the well-known band Dropkick Murphy's). In the scene on the shirt, people are shown toting signs that read "United We Bargain!" and "Divided We Beg!"

"I got to meet him and talk to him on a personal level and he told me, 'Veterans helping veterans is the key,'" Jake says. The seeds were planted for what has become Jake's life's work and passion: connecting vets with cannabis. He started a program at the collective where he worked that donated medicine to veterans, and partnered with two fellow military returnees who grew marijuana for the dispensary.

In 2014, he left that job and moved about an hour south to the woodsy hamlet of Bonny Doon, in Santa Cruz County, to work with those growers at their organization, the Santa Cruz Veterans Alliance (scveteransalliance.com). As manager of its Veterans Compassion Program, Jake helped grow the membership from 10 to 50 participants, who come together about twice a month to socialize, partake in activities like ocean kayaking, and receive free cannabis medicine.

Life since the move "has been pretty good," Jake says with a grin that suggests this is an understatement.

He's still fighting a battle all too familiar to veterans. Slamming doors, loud noises, someone standing too close behind him in a line—life is full of triggers, but they no longer overwhelm him.

"[PTSD] is still very much part of my life," he says. "There are good days and bad days. Cannabis lets me handle the triggers, allows me acknowledge them."

"You're not on medication anymore, either," Effie adds. The physical act of growing and tending a marijuana garden, which he also does for the Santa Cruz Veterans Alliance, has bolstered his wellbeing, helping him shed 35 pounds and practice patience and mindfulness.

Effie grows teary eyed as she describes Jake's progress over the last four years.

"I've really seen the whole transformation, the 180 [degree change]," she says. "It's like night and day. It's phenomenal. Cannabis has allowed him to be present and I'm thankful for that. That's why we're pushing for this [veteran access to cannabis], because if it can happen for him, it can happen for anybody. So, as long as the need is there, we'll be there, too."

Bandit chimes in with a few quick barks, alerting his owners that another dog has just entered the patio. Jake soothes him and tells him it's OK. The dog jumps onto the bench, taking a watchful post between the husband-and-wife to be.

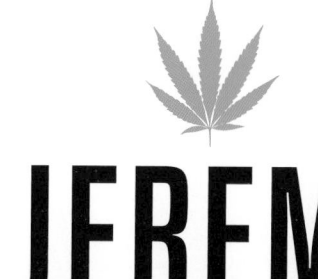

JEREMY BOURQUE

Age 38 / **Frontal Lobe Nocturnal Epilepsy** / Port Arthur, Texas

One morning, not long after Jeremy Bourque was attacked by a group of people "looking for trouble," the then-15-year-old didn't wake up.

Jeremy's parents took him to the hospital, where a doctor declared that he had an aneurism. It had actually been a seizure—the first of many that followed as a result of injuries incurred by the attack—but it would be years before Jeremy knew the truth about his condition.

"For 15 years [doctors] were trying to tell me I was having bad dreams, and that's why I was waking up with black eyes and having punched myself," he says.

The years of medical unhelpfulness were frustrating, and also increasingly dangerous.

"When I was younger, it was easier to get over having a seizure—my body

recovered more easily," he says. "As I started getting older and having more, it became a lot harder." The episodes would cause him to forget everything that happened in the preceding days, and required two or three additional days of recuperation afterward.

Jeremy resorted to conducting his own research and used the findings to convince his doctors to test him for epilepsy, leading finally to a diagnosis of frontal lobe nocturnal epilepsy in 2002. His studies also brought his attention to cannabis as a treatment. When he tried it, he slept through the night and awoke unscathed. "I didn't have black eyes," he says.

Jeremy began growing marijuana in 1995, producing nine months' worth of medicine from just three or four plants. He has used cannabis, both by smoking it

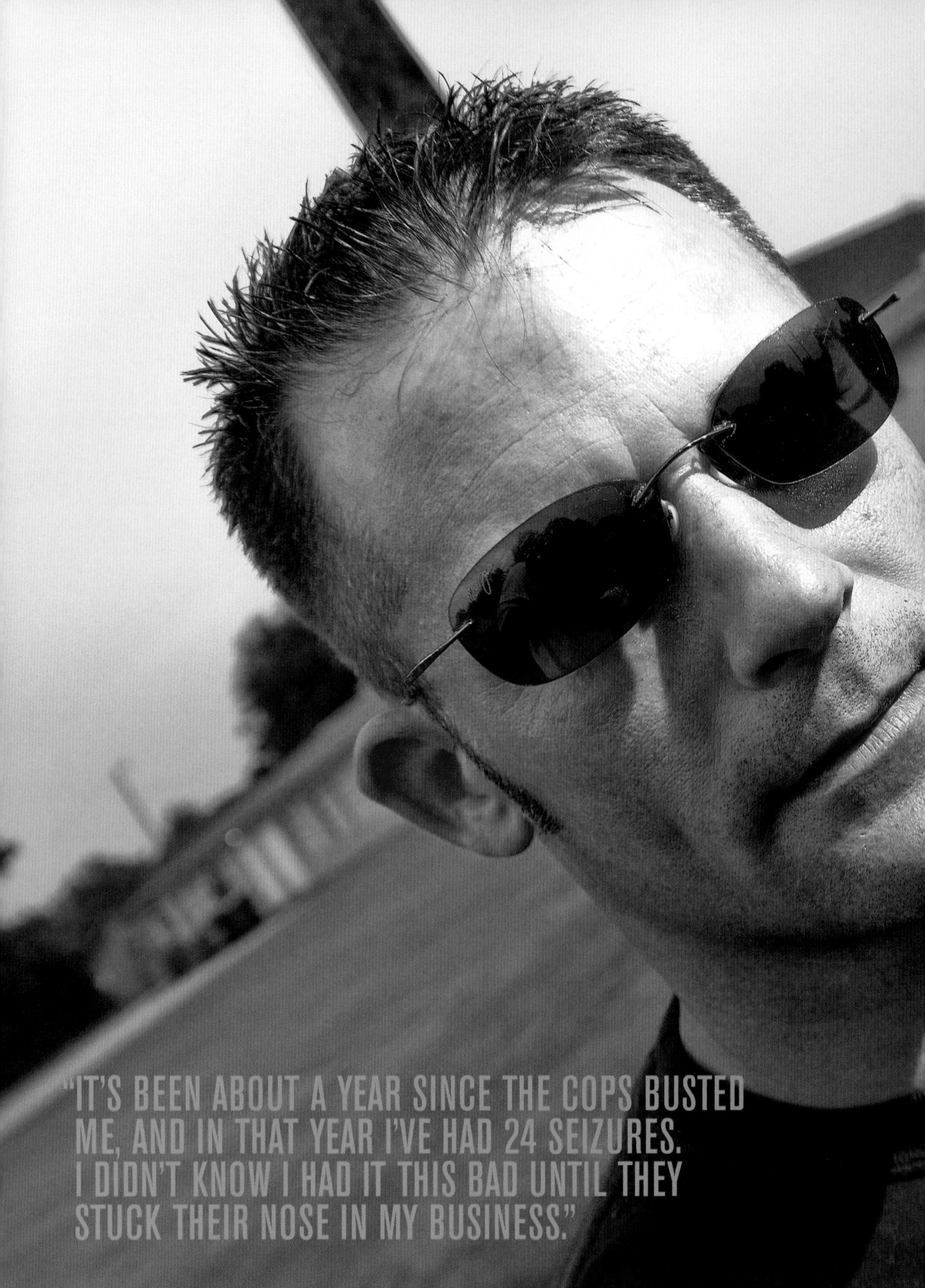

"IT'S BEEN ABOUT A YEAR SINCE THE COPS BUSTED ME, AND IN THAT YEAR I'VE HAD 24 SEIZURES. I DIDN'T KNOW I HAD IT THIS BAD UNTIL THEY STUCK THEIR NOSE IN MY BUSINESS."

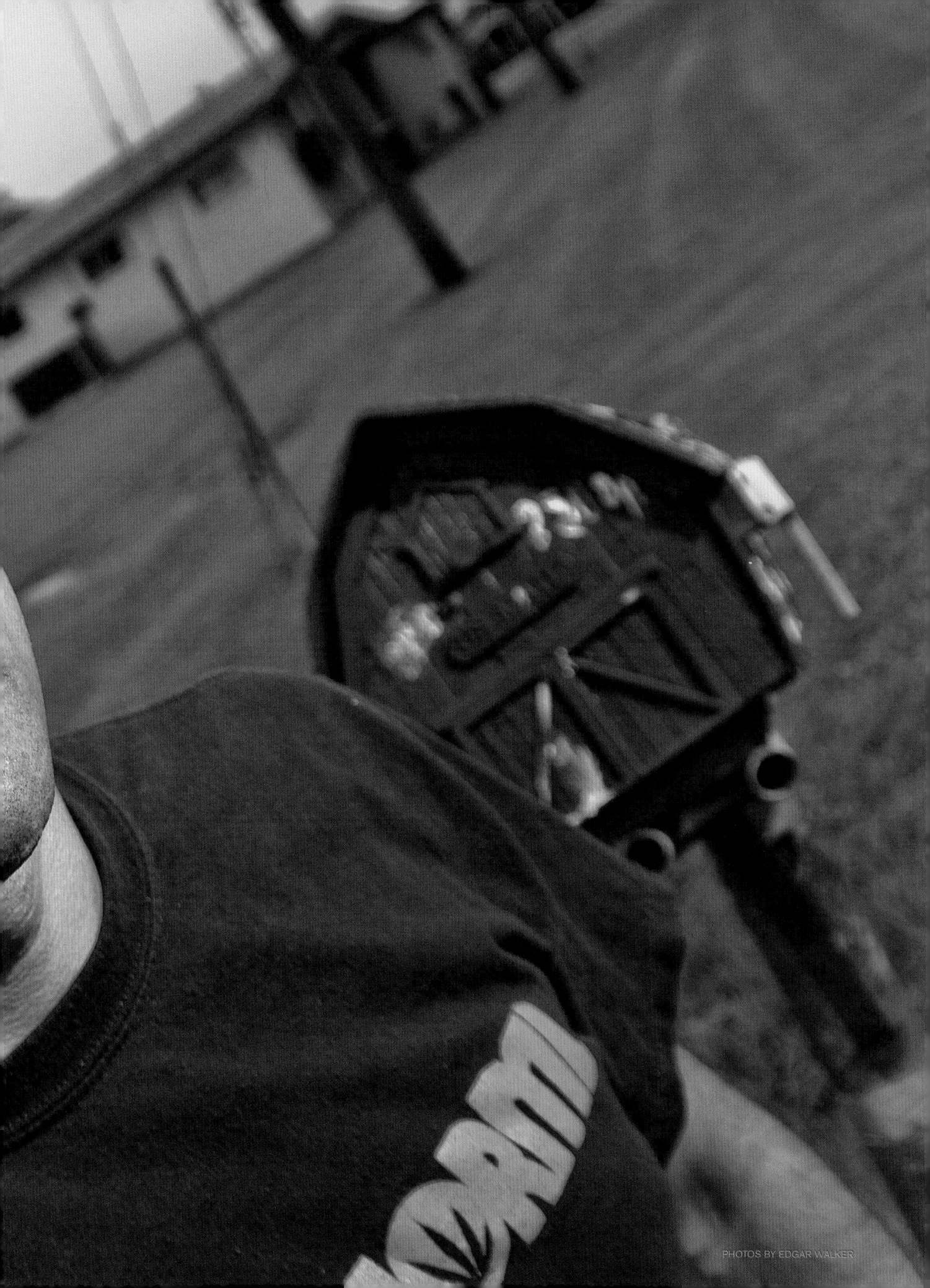

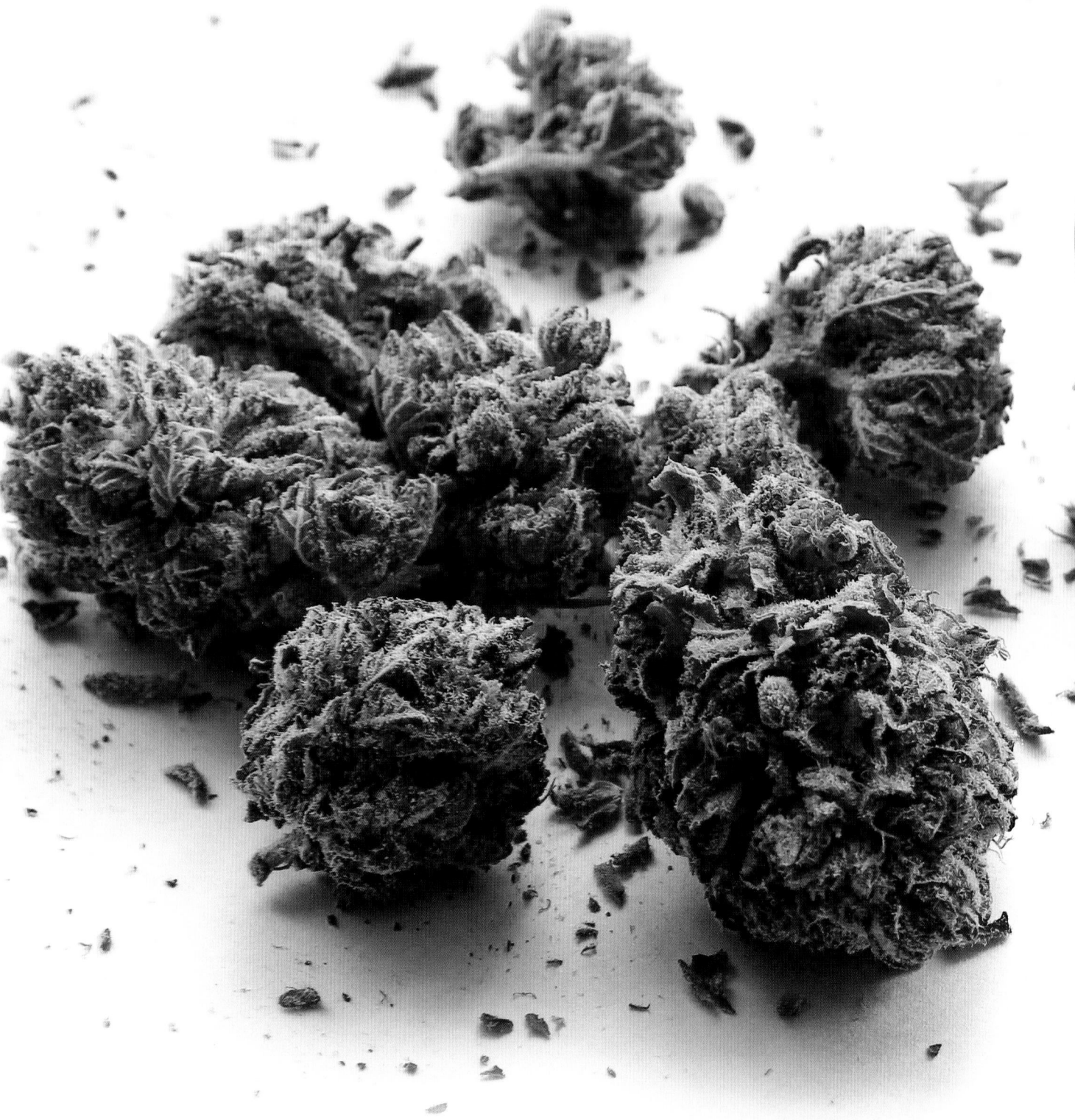

WHERE STATES STAND: Twenty-three states plus Washington, D.C., currently have medical marijuana laws, according to the National Conference of State Legislatures. An additional 15 states allow limited use of CBD oil for medicinal use or as a legal defense. So far, Colorado, Washington, Oregon, Alaska and Washington, D.C., have legalized marijuana for recreational use, according to NORML.

As of this writing, Pennsylvania has a measure to legalize medical marijuana pending a vote, while 17 other states introduced but failed to pass medical marijuana laws in 2015, according to ProCon.org. The United States Congress is also considering one piece of legislation that would remove low-THC concentrations of cannabis from the federal definition of marijuana, and another that would move marijuana off Schedule I of the Controlled Substances Act entirely.

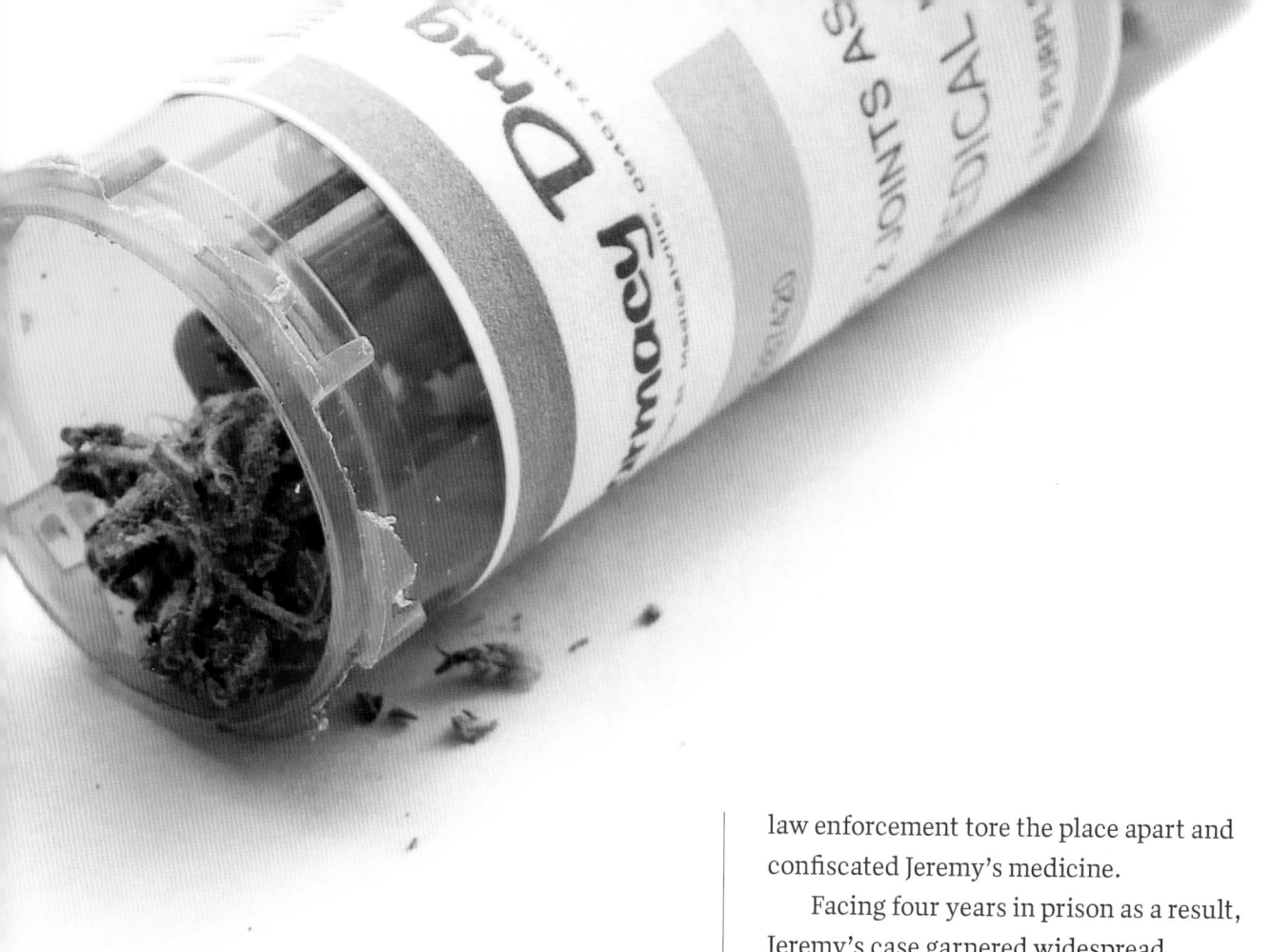

and ingesting oils, for more than 20 years, with empowering results. However, he does so in Texas, which did not have any form of medical cannabis law until June 2015 (when the governor signed a law that legalized the use of CBD strains for treating certain types of epilepsy), and does not have the financial means to relocate to a state that is more accommodating to patients. He's faced the consequences of that as a result. In 2014, Jeremy, who works as a residential and commercial painter, was on a job about 20 miles away from the home he shares with his grandmother, whom he takes care of. She was home alone when law enforcement tore the place apart and confiscated Jeremy's medicine.

Facing four years in prison as a result, Jeremy's case garnered widespread attention and support. "I was hoping that they would take it to trial and that people would see that I was doing what I had to do to stay alive. If I did go to prison, it would just be a matter of time until I shook myself to death. I'd flail, break my nose, give myself black eyes, and bite my tongue off."

As of this writing, the case was on the trial docket, but a date had yet to be set. Jeremy continues to use cannabis—it's a matter of life or death, he says—but now must find it on the black market. When he grew his own, he rotated between six different strains and had excellent results. "It's been about a year since the cops busted me, and in that year I've had 24 seizures," he says. "I didn't know I had it this bad until they stuck their nose in my business."

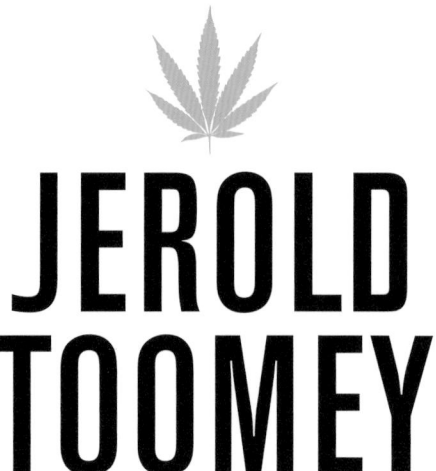

JEROLD TOOMEY

Age 67 / **Acute Full Body Tendonitis** / Cleveland, Ohio

Full-body tendonitis hit Jerold Toomey in 1999 with no clear cause.

"I worked as a toolmaker in machining, and all kinds of industries that use chemicals and Lord knows what—they didn't tell us," the 67-year-old Ohioan says. "I don't know where the tendonitis came from, perhaps from handling cold steel." Another contributor might have been an accident that year, in which he fell off a 10-speed bike.

By 2001, he was bedridden, victim to an inflamed, protesting body. His ability to carry out basic tasks diminished. "I had pain-induced amnesia," he says. "That's how severe my pain was. It wiped out my mind. I struggled to remember my name. I had to concentrate before I could give it."

The inability to cook for himself—a passion he formed while working the grill as a short-order cook in high school and, later, at a steakhouse he ran with his brothers—was particularly heart wrenching. Even boiling water became too complicated; he just burned the pan. Needless to say, he could no longer work, and was on disability. His girlfriend, with whom he has an autistic son, cared for him.

Meanwhile, Jerold, a Vietnam War veteran, got "the runaround" from the VA, which misdiagnosed him with bone cancer. "They never investigated anything. They just started treating me with pain pills that didn't do much at all," he says.

He took the advice of friends and family and tried smoking marijuana to curb the pain. The inhalation of THC

"IF IT WASN'T FOR THC, THE TENDONITIS WOULD NOT HAVE ABATED AND I'D BE DEAD. I COULDN'T MOVE. IT WAS GETTING TO WHERE I COULDN'T EVEN BREATHE. IT CHANGED MY LIFE."

quickly proved to be the only thing that helped. "I remember that first puff so well," he says. "It was the first time in months that I could stand up straight."

Overall, he says THC reduced the severity of his condition and made it tolerable.

"It worked. It got me out of bed," he says. "If it wasn't for THC, the tendonitis would not have abated and I'd be dead. I couldn't move. It was getting to where I couldn't even breathe. It changed my life."

But Jerold lives in Cleveland, in a state that has not yet legalized medical marijuana. In September 2008, he was pulled over on his way home from buying his black-market medicine and ticketed. At the resulting court date, the judge deemed that Jerold attend Alcoholics Anonymous and an alcohol assessment and treatment program—frustrating punishment for Jerold, who does not drink. Living on the limited means of disability checks, he couldn't afford transportation to the meetings and had to walk through the frost and ice of an Ohio winter in order to attend. "Tendonitis is a serious death threat in the cold weather," he says.

Despite the risks, Jerold continues to use THC because of the benefits it has brought him. Among those, it gave him enough pain relief to do the hard work necessary to recover his memories.

Jerold's son Gareth, now 24, took charge of this task, determined to help his father recover his short- and long-term memory. Over the course of several years, Gareth would sit Jerold down and grill him about his past, particularly about his time as a toolmaker and machinist.

"My son is autistic and has this kind of energy when he wants to," Jerold says. "He only made it through fifth grade but he's self-taught in many fields. It was so interesting to observe how he picked my brain expertly about my experiences in the machining field. ... I would describe a memory, [then] he would research it online and come back with more tough questions that forced me to concentrate deeper."

The process felt "like I was going through soul surgery in the hands of the divine," says Jerold.

After years of not being able to cook, or even make coffee, Jerold is in the kitchen again. "I'm back to cooking. In fact," he says, "I just made bread today."

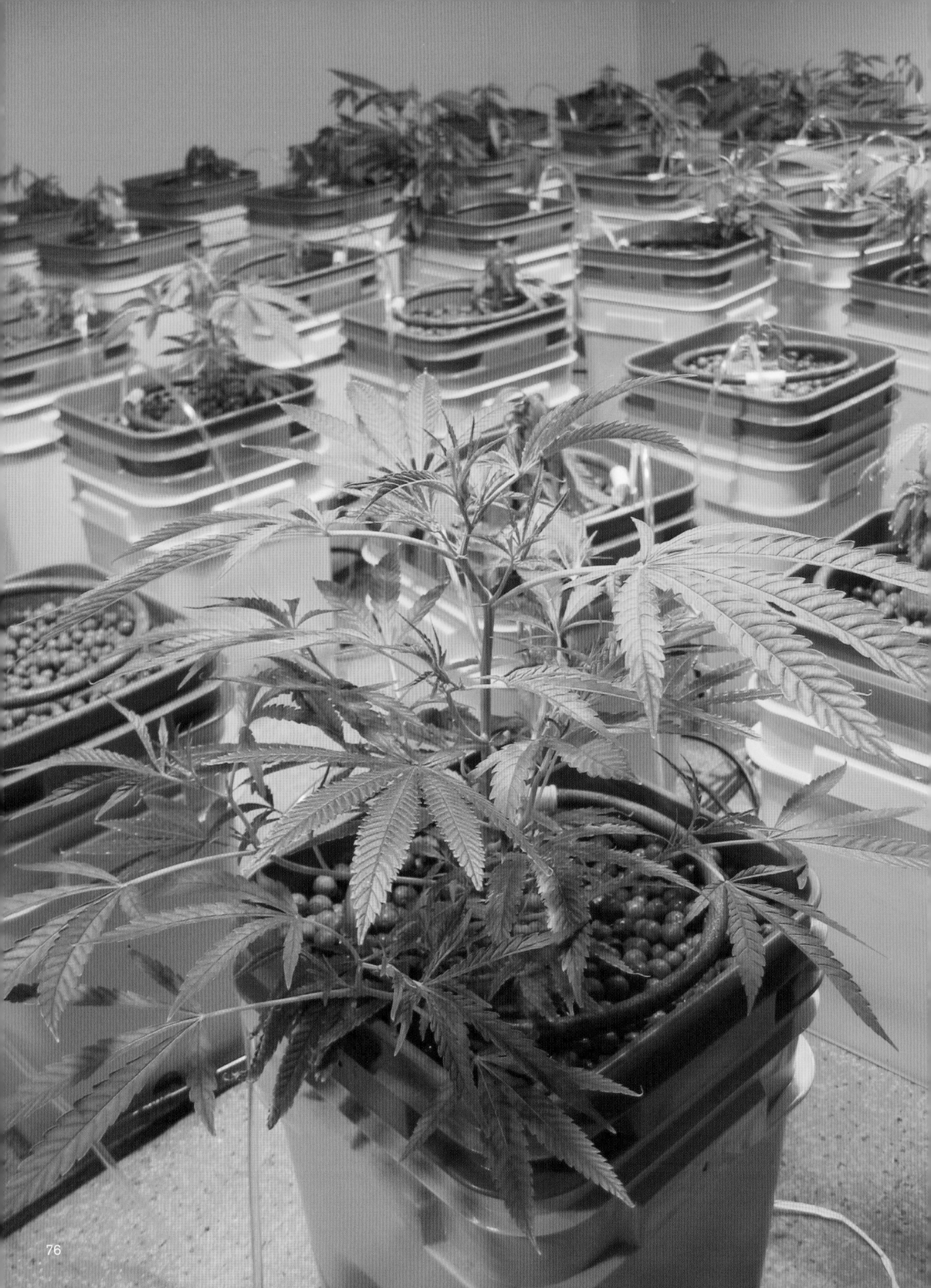

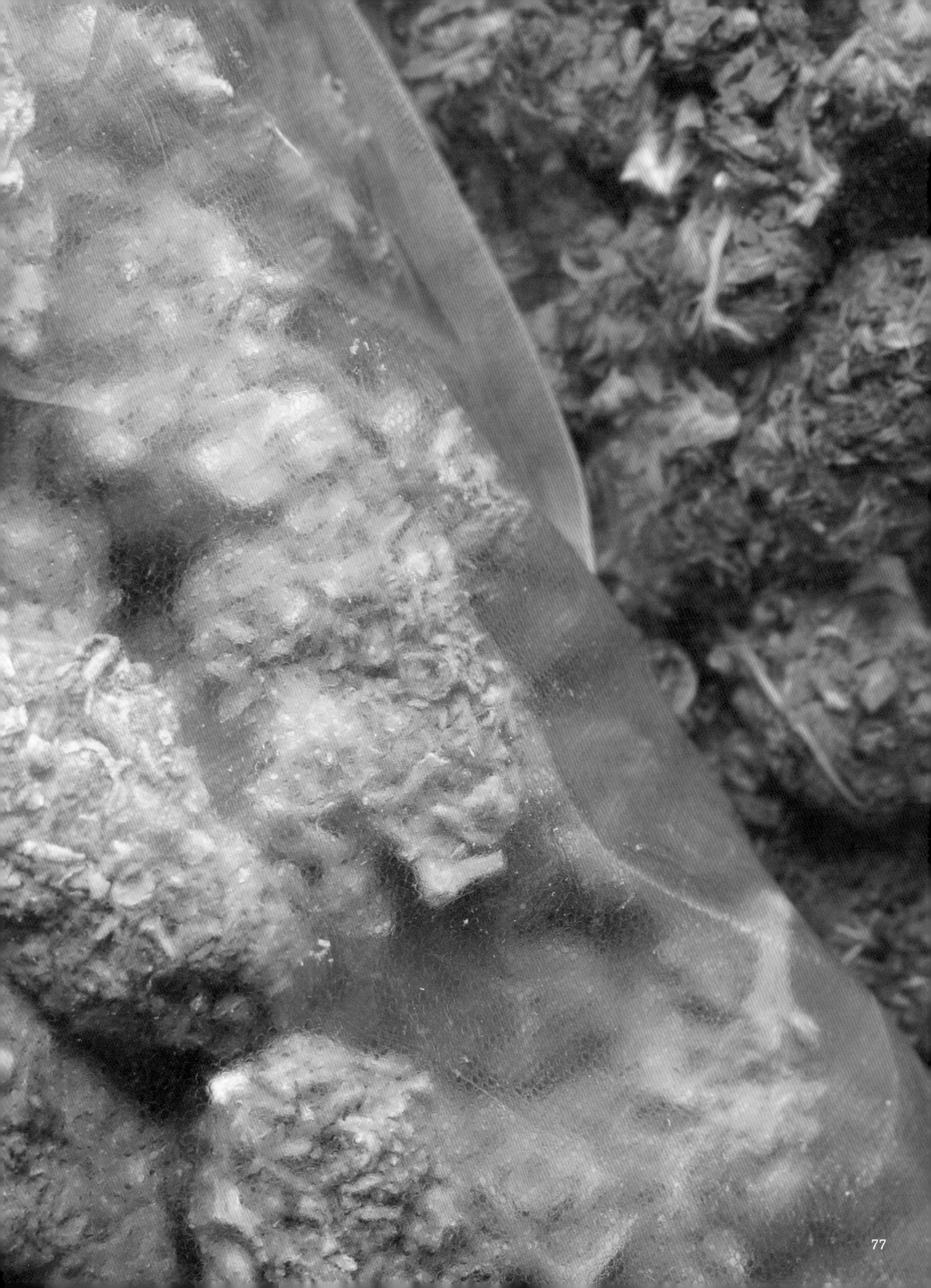

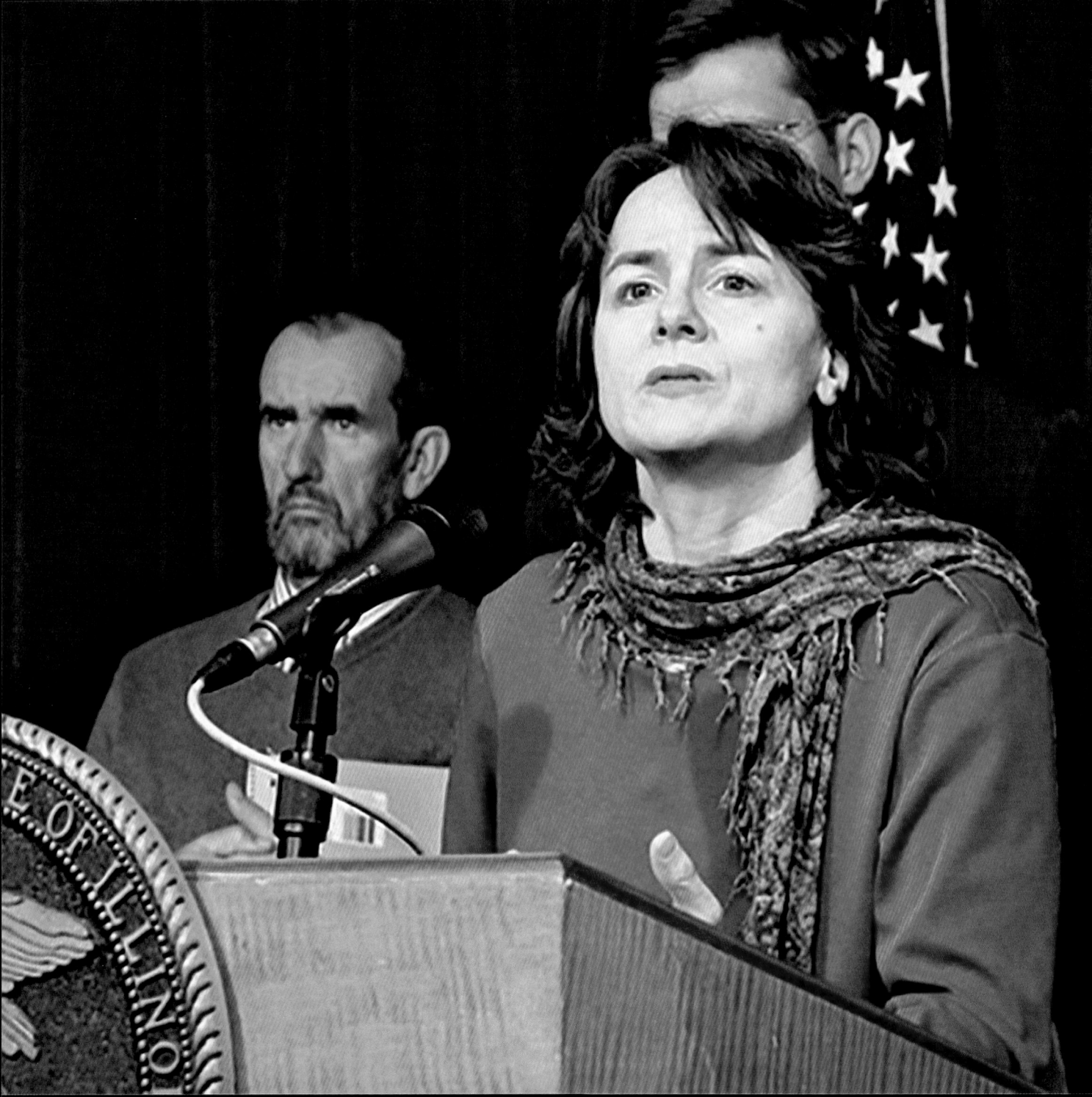

"IF WE ARE IN THE DEEPEST, DARKEST PLACE ... THERE IS ALWAYS SOME LITTLE SLIVER OF HOPE, SOMETHING ELSE TO TRY."

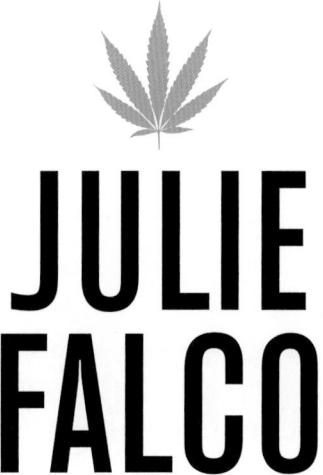

JULIE FALCO

Age 50 / **Multiple Sclerosis** / Chicago, Illinois

In 1986, while a third-year communications major at Illinois State University, Julie Falco spent spring break at home in South Holland, Illinois, lounging and resting and waiting for the small wedding ceremony in which her mother would be remarried.

When she interrupted her R&R with a trip to the grocery store, she was puzzled to discover that her left foot wasn't cooperating. Her toes dragged on the ground as she walked from the car to the market. Did I pinch a nerve?, she wondered. Was I too lazy hanging around the house?

The family chiropractor ran several tests and, unsure of what the problem might be, requested that Julie stick around for further testing. But school beckoned, as did her band—an alternative outfit in the order of The Cure and

Talking Heads called Zero Balance—so she left after the wedding, a modest service at her grandmother's house.

The left side of her body was tingly and numb, but she went forward with playing the band's scheduled gigs. At the first performance, Julie, who is right-handed, noticed her left arm and leg felt "off" so she sat on a barstool while she played guitar. The next performance didn't go as well: part way through the set, Julie motioned to her band that she could no longer play and went to sit down. Her arm had gone stiff and froze in a bent position at the elbow, and the prickly sensation she had felt before was heightened. Her band mates took her to an emergency room when the show was over, where she stayed overnight to have a series of tests done. Doctors thought it could be multiple sclerosis (MS), but weren't sure. They scheduled her for a spinal tap a week later.

"By the time I went in for the appointment a week later, I'd slept the whole week and everything was fine," Julie remembers. "Everything had subsided. I regained movement in my arm and leg."

Two years went by without any problems. The MS scare was fading into the past when, in 1988, Julie's eyesight temporarily vanished and her face was partially paralyzed. She was then officially diagnosed with MS, a disease in which "damage to the myelin coating around the nerve fibers … interferes with the transmission of nerve signals between the brain, spinal cord and the rest of the body," according to the National Multiple Sclerosis Society.

Julie's neurologist, suffering from a lack of bedside manner, handed her a book about the disease and said, "There's not much you can do." His defeated attitude wasn't unjust; there simply wasn't the understanding of or support for MS then that there is now, Julie explains.

As the years progressed, so did Julie's condition. At first, her MS manifested as minor limping—"an odd gait to my step," she says. Her left foot began to drag more noticeably, and the numbness and tingling worsened. Eventually she needed a cane to walk, and then two canes, and then a walker to get around her apartment. Today, she is able to stand but does not walk normally. "I can't put one foot in front of the other," she says. Once she pulls herself up with the aid of grab bars, her feet stubbornly solid and unmoving on the ground, she does a sliding motion, swishing side to side. For longer distances, she relies on a wheelchair.

As for music, she was able to play in bands for another three years after her diagnosis, and play some guitar until 2010, when it became too difficult to hold the strings down. While the condition is still concentrated mostly on her left side, it began distributing "across both sides at varying degrees," she says.

The advancing symptoms depressed Julie. By the time the millennium came to a close, she was unable to work full time—she had worked for a theatrical lighting company and a phone company—and began cobbling together odd jobs that she could do from home. She took all of the medications suggested by her doctors, including muscle relaxers, an injectable drug, and prescriptions for depression and muscle spasticity. She was lethargic and dejected. She lacked motivation and energy. And she thought it was all due to the MS.

"I wanted to sleep all the time, and that led to more depression," she says. "I thought it was just going to get worse."

What she didn't realize was that a lot of her symptoms were actually side effects from prescriptions. The situation grew dourer until, in 2004, Julie considered ending it all with suicide.

"I thought, 'This isn't a quality of life I am interested in, and I don't want to subject anyone in my family to it,'" she says. "I thought, 'It's just going to get worse until I lose all functionality, until I can't feed and bath myself.' I was under a very heavy dark cloud."

As a last-ditch effort, Julie tried baking cannabis into brownies. She had previously found that smoking marijuana helped reduce her muscle spasms, but it aggravated her headaches, which she was prone to getting. Right away, the brownies made a difference, reducing leg spasticity, improving walking abilities, abating her insomnia and depression, and helping control her bladder. "I was amazed at how it was working for me and that it had no side effects that I could see," she says.

The brownies became part of Julie's treatment routine alongside the pharmaceuticals, until she weaned herself off of everything else in 2007.

As is the case for so many sick and suffering cannabis patients in states with prohibitive laws, Julie dealt with the troubles of having to obtain illegal marijuana until 2013, when Illinois passed a medical marijuana bill. Although her physical limitations would have made it extremely difficult, Julie came so close in the interim years to ditching Illinois for a legal state that she packed all of her belongings.

She spends much of her time spreading her story, doing research, and connecting with others about the medical value of cannabis. "I talk to people with MS, Parkinson's, cancer, glaucoma—you name it. Friends and other people pass them along to talk to me about their options. They've run out of help from pharmaceuticals."

Throughout her advocacy, Julie has made a conscious decision to rid her vocabulary of the "M word."

"I don't use the term marijuana—it's a demonized term," she says, pointing to its popularization during the 20th century debates that brought about the plant's prohibition. "I had doors shut in my face when I said 'medical marijuana' … I realized [advocates] aren't going to get anywhere this way, and that we need to start calling it what it is in a medical term if we're going to get any kind of attention. Now I say 'medical cannabis' and it gets me in the door and gets conversations started."

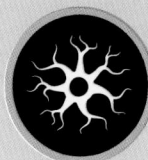

MS: Multiple sclerosis, or MS, is a disease that occurs when the immune system reacts against the central nervous system, damaging the brain's ability to send and receive information to and from the body. Extensive scientific evidence shows that cannabis can help control pain and other symptoms associated with MS, and some studies suggest that the plant can limit the progression of the disease. *Sources: National Multiple Sclerosis Society, NORML.*

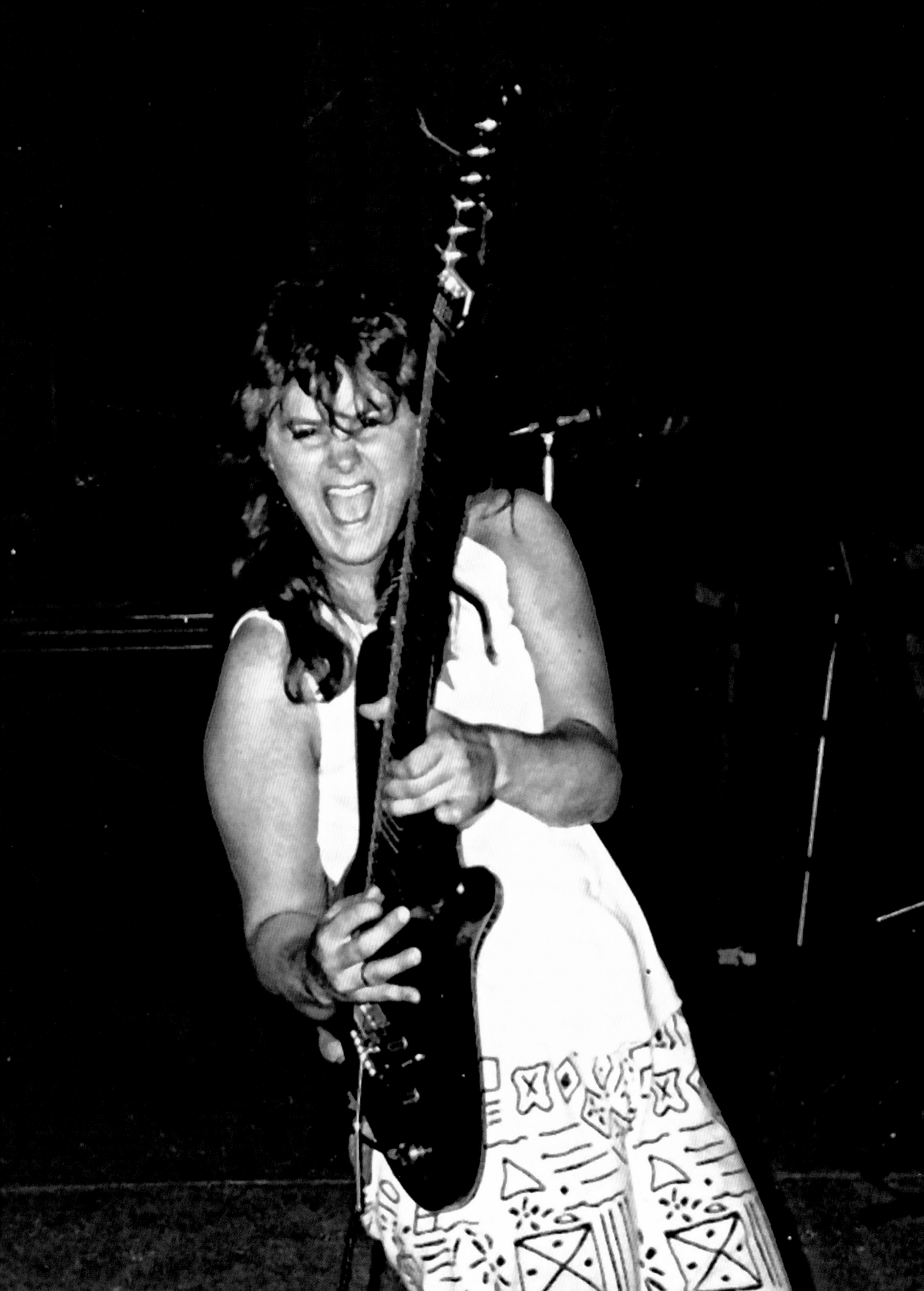

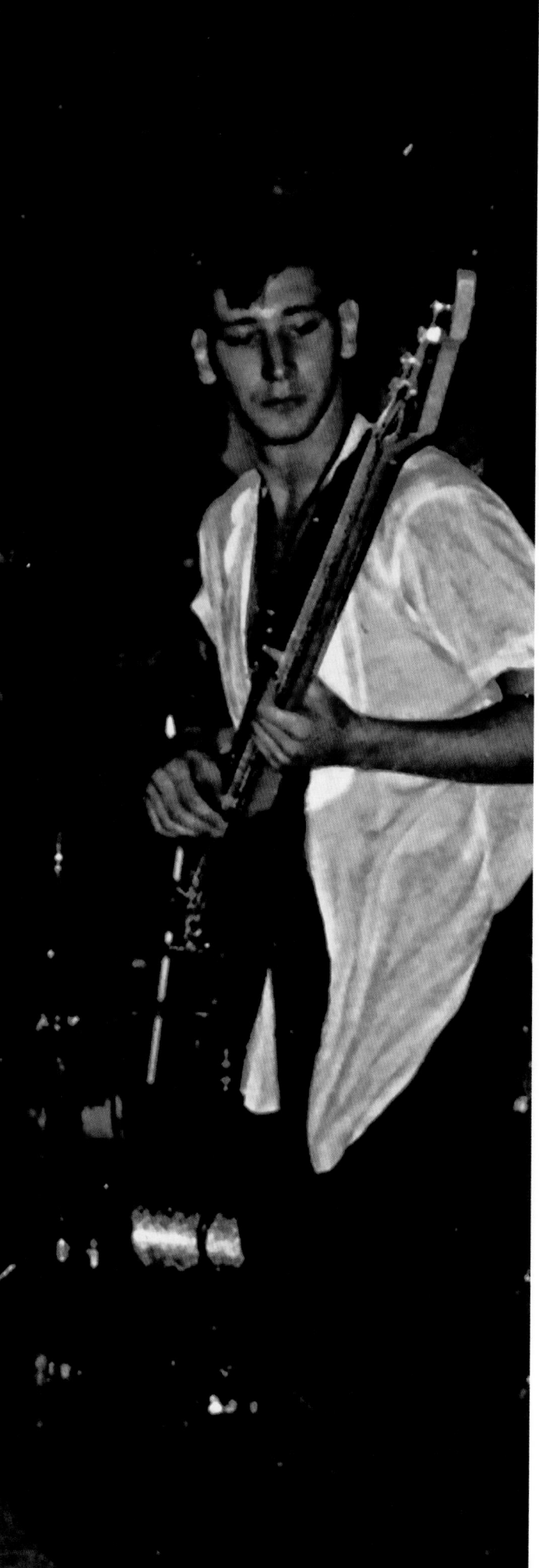

"I THOUGHT 'IT'S JUST GOING TO GET WORSE UNTIL I LOSE ALL FUNCTIONALITY, UNTIL I CAN'T FEED AND BATH MYSELF.' I WAS UNDER A VERY HEAVY DARK CLOUD."

Returning it to its proper name, and away from a word entrenched in constructed stereotypes and fears, is one way she believes perceptions of the plant can be shifted into the more positive light it deserves.

"It's taking care of the majority of all of the symptoms that I deal with concerning the MS," she says. "Next year it will be 30 years [of MS], and I do have medical staff and people who do home visits who are astounded that I've had it for so long and am doing great. I give a lot of props to cannabis. My message for others is that if we are in the deepest, darkest place ... there is always some little sliver of hope, something else to try."

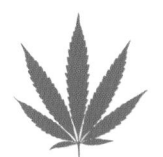

LAURA MASTROPIETRO

Age 50 / **Porphyria** / Sedona, Arizona

The Hideaway House restaurant in Sedona, Arizona, is perched on a lush hillside above a creek, with double-decker balconies that offer views of the iconic red rock formations jutting into the Southwestern sky.

Behind the kitchen doors is Steve Schnirch, the chef, and behind other aspects of the business is his wife, Laura Mastropietro, who runs the place and also makes desserts. The couple opened the eatery in June 2014, having taken it over from previous ownership and reinvented it. They are transplants from Phoenix, where Laura sprouted a passion for baking while making cannabis brownies for a medical marijuana co-op and, later, bakeries.

Running a restaurant is a laborious process, and one that would not be possible for Laura were it not for cannabis, which she uses to manage symptoms of porphyria, a rare condition she was diagnosed with in 2004.

Pronounced poor-FEAR-e-uh, it is actually a grouping of differing disorders that, in simple terms, can create problems with the body's nervous system, skin and other organs. Musing on porphyria's scarcity—it affects fewer than 200,000 Americans, according to porphyriafoundation.com—Laura thinks of a surgeon in his 60s who frequents the Hideaway House. "I'm the first one he's ever met," Laura says. "And he's met a lot of medically interesting people."

Her health issues arose in the late '90s, when one half of her face would sometimes go numb down the side of her nose, lip and cheek. After a trip to the ER

"I'M GETTING PHONE CALLS FROM PEOPLE ALL OVER THE COUNTRY WHO HAVE HEARD THERE IS NOTHING MORE THAT CAN BE DONE FOR THEM, THAT THEY NEED TO WAIT IT OUT AND PASS AWAY."

in 1999, she was misdiagnosed with a brain tumor and put on Dilantin, an anti-convulsant with warnings that include "liver damage" and "an increased risk of suicidal thoughts," for the three weeks it was believed she had a tumor.

It was the start of a long and tiring saga of misdiagnoses and medical puzzlement, persisting until she was finally diagnosed with porphyria five years later. In the first nine months following the brain tumor slipup, doctors thought her problem might be stress-induced chronic fatigue and skin cancer (it took 12 skin-punch biopsies to find out it wasn't), and

removed her gall bladder to address abdominal pain.

Meanwhile, her symptoms heightened. At random, she would go temporarily blind, or paralyzed from the neck down. She struggled to keep food down for the entire five years of the health mystery.

"They scoped and prodded," she says. "They ruled out Lupus. They ruled out gut issues. They were pretty sure it was atypical MS at the end of the five years."

A longtime social worker, Laura resigned to long-term disability and living out her years without answers and in significant pain. "It felt like broken glass inside my bones," she says. For the year

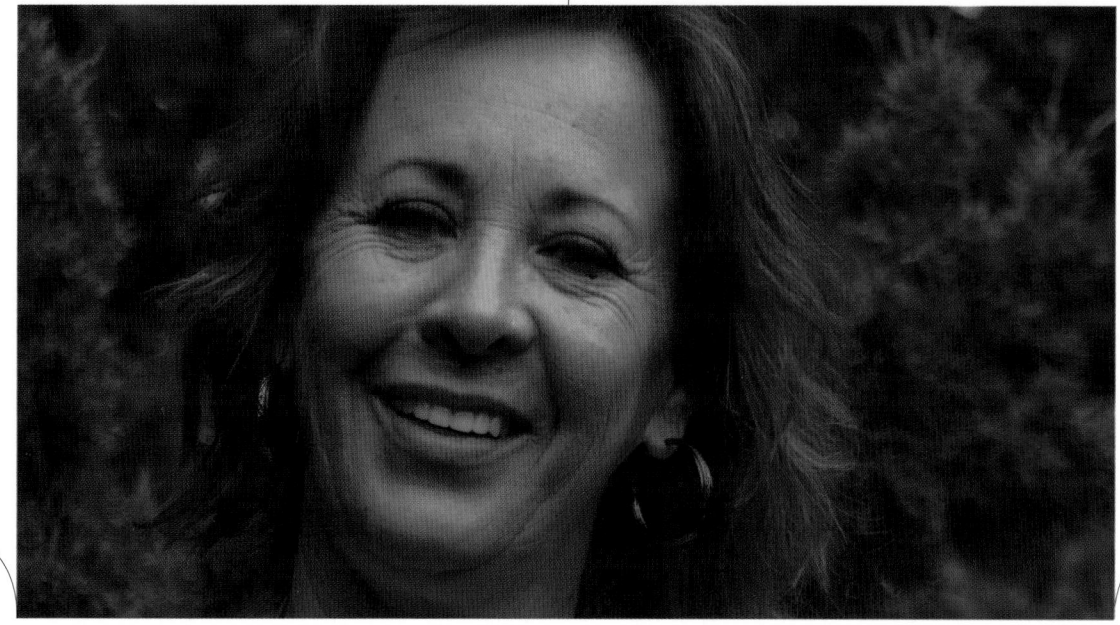

leading up to her diagnosis, she had to take the narcotic pain reliever Demerol four times daily just to be capable of standing or walking. "And I hate pain pills—when I'm on them, I tell all my secrets," she says.

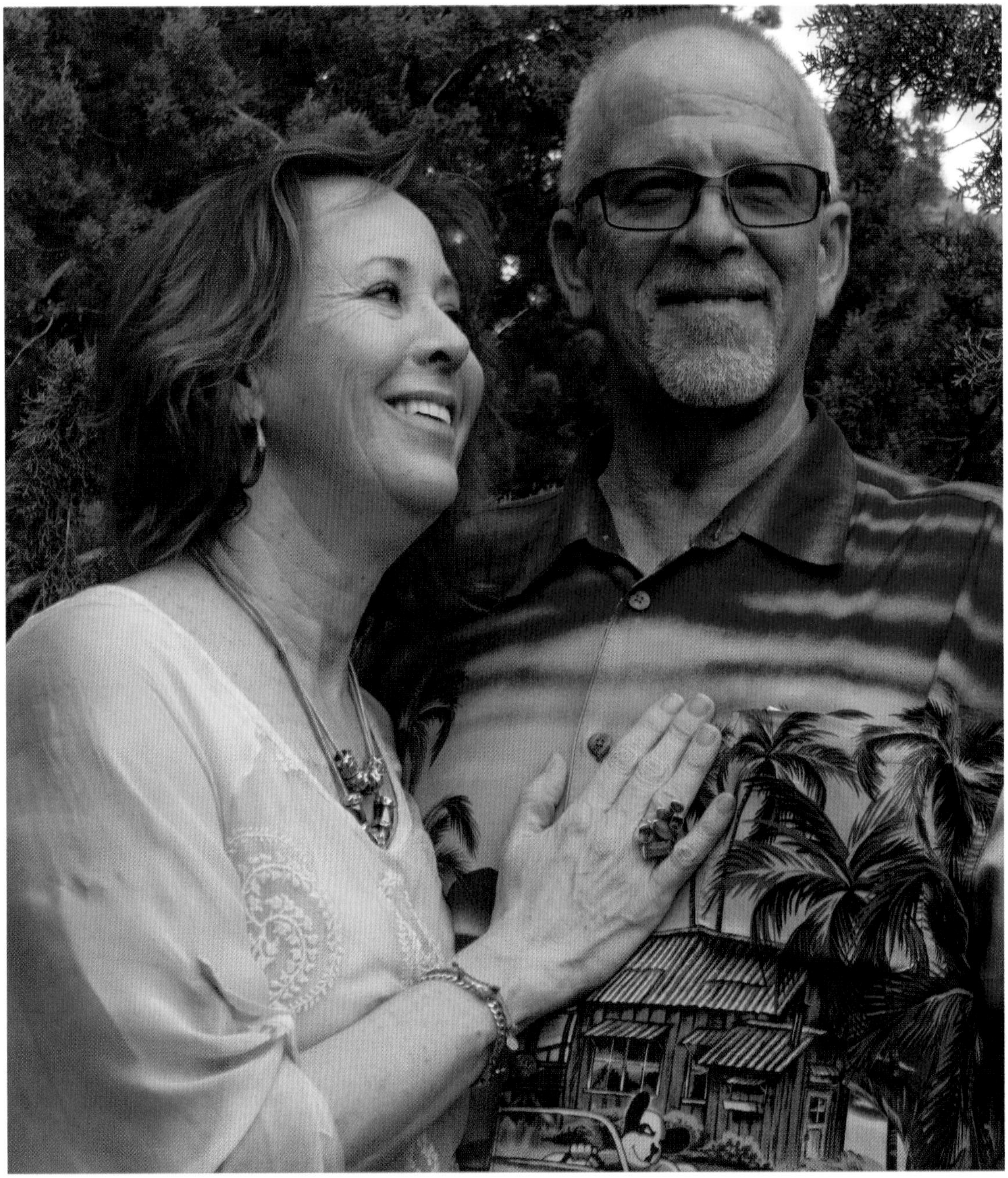

Unbeknownst to Laura and her doctors, the treatments were exacerbating her actual condition, which was fueled by neurotoxic buildup from the drugs. "Medications were the worst thing for the disorder," she adds. "Every drug for every symptom over the years activated the sleeping monster of porphyria, aggravating the condition and causing a new set of symptoms."

Finally, in 2004, Laura was officially diagnosed with porphyria. Being diagnosed with an uncommon and incurable disease is never good news, but it did mean Laura finally had some answers. "It's kind of like a race, where you're at the finish line and you honestly don't think you'll make it, you won't finish, then you get that little burst in your sails, like you're going to finish … knowing, 'I'm not going to die.'"

Six months later, Laura and Steve—her "superhero husband," whom she'd first moved in with around the time of that misdiagnosed brain tumor—were married in Greece and honeymooned in Venice. By the time they returned, Laura was gaunt and sickly looking. She began treatment immediately—a 24/7 intravenous glucose drip, which porphyriafoundation.com explains "can prevent an attack or can hasten recovery from an attack of the acute porphyrias." Her pain was gone within four days. Although she still has flare-ups, hooking up to one of the many sugar-water IVs she has stationed around her home takes the pain level "from a monster to an annoyance."

Through it all, she has turned to cannabis for physical and emotional relief. "I used it the whole time I was sick along with the pain meds," she says. "It helped with nausea. It kept me off of anti-depressants [and] probably off of suicide watch. I used to call it 'smoking a little hope.' There were a lot of days … when [the pain is such that] you can't move off your floor for 20 minutes. The anti-depressant values of using cannabis are extremely undervalued. It significantly helps with your outlook on life."

Since Arizona passed a medical cannabis law in 2010, Laura (now a legal patient) uses only cannabis and glucose for treatment, and she lives a high-functioning, active life. She speaks to a lot of women who deal with issues similar to hers—many of whom she says are mistakenly told they have chronic pain. She's currently in the process of developing a cannabis-consulting network. She wants to teach suffering people that they can medicate without becoming a "stoner stereotype"—that they don't have to smoke if they prefer not to; that they can even drink a dose of cannabis in their morning cup of coffee and go on to have a pain-free day.

"I'm getting phone calls from people all over the country who have heard there is nothing more that can be done for them, that they need to wait it out and pass away," Laura says. "People from states where it's not legal. They are coming from a place of having never smelled pot except maybe one time when they walked past their brother's bedroom. They need someone to hold their hands."

She's happy to be that someone.

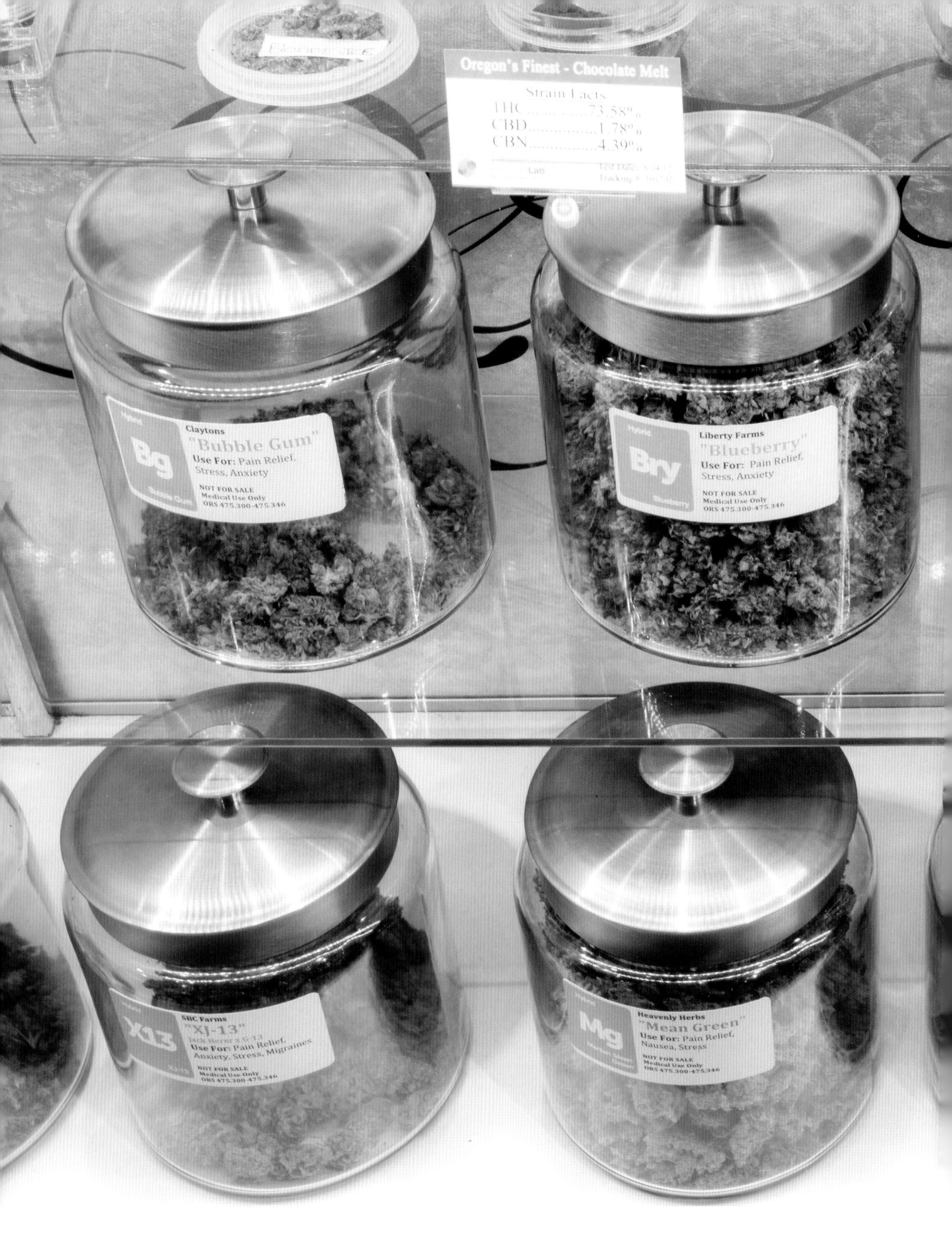

88

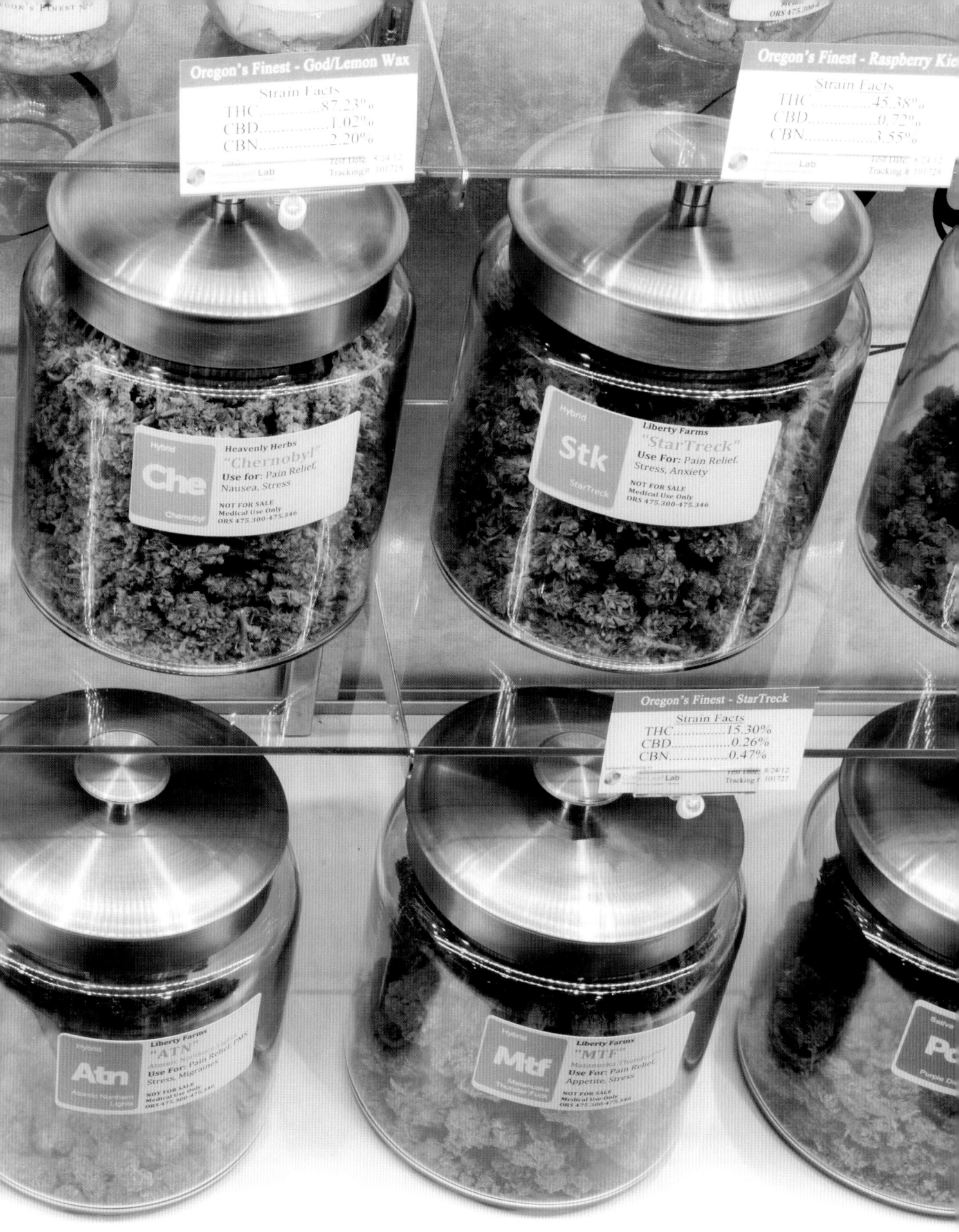

Oregon's Finest - God/Lemon Wax

Strain Facts

THC................87.23%
CBD.................1.02%
CBN................2.20%

Lab

Test Date: 8/24/12
Tracking# 101725

Oregon's Finest - Raspberry Kie...

Strain Facts

THC................45.38%
CBD.................0.72%
CBN................3.55%

Lab

Test Date: 8/24/12
Tracking # 101728

Hybrid

Che

Chernobyl

Heavenly Herbs

"Chernobyl"
Use for: Pain Relief,
Nausea, Stress

NOT FOR SALE
Medical Use Only
ORS 475.300-475.346

Hybrid

Stk

StarTreck

Liberty Farms

"StarTreck"
Use For: Pain Relief,
Stress, Anxiety

NOT FOR SALE
Medical Use Only
ORS 475.300-475.346

Oregon's Finest - StarTreck

Strain Facts

THC................15.30%
CBD.................0.26%
CBN................0.47%

Lab

Test Date: 8/24/12
Tracking # 101727

Hybrid

Atn

Alaskan Northern Lights

Liberty Farms

"ATN"
Use For: Pain Relief,
Stress, Migraines

NOT FOR SALE
Medical Use Only
ORS 475.300-475.346

Hybrid

Mtf

Matanuska Thunderfuck

Liberty Farms

"MTF"
Use For: Pain Relief,
Appetite, Stress

NOT FOR SALE
Medical Use Only
ORS 475.300-475.346

Po

Purple Dr...

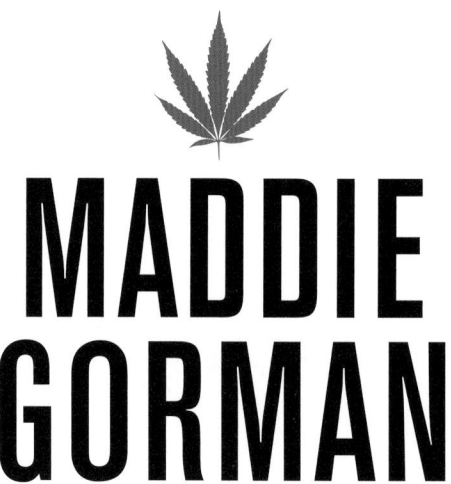

MADDIE GORMAN

Age 8 / **Infant Leukemia, Epilepsy** / Colorado Springs, Colorado

"**C**an I call you back in three minutes? I need to get my daughter on the potty."

In these matter-of-fact introductory words, Liz Gorman's voice is staggeringly upbeat, which surprises me. Back on the phone a few minutes later, Liz relays the details of her 8-year-old daughter Maddie's battle with infant leukemia and epilepsy.

"I'm a naturally optimistic person," Liz says. "I felt like my poor kid couldn't have been brought here to Earth to suffer like this. She had cancer, then severe epilepsy. I always had great hope that something was going to work."

After a lifetime marked by chemotherapy, dangerous seizures, a baker's dozen of tried-and-failed anti-epileptic pharmaceuticals and treatments, and

brain surgery, Maddie is, for the first time, not just surviving but thriving.

That "something" that eventually worked was Charlotte's Web, a liquid cannabis extract made in Colorado that is high in cannabidiol (CBD, an active cannabinoid with wide medical applications) and low in tetrahydrocannabinol (or THC, the main psychoactive component in cannabis), and is used to treat epilepsy in children. Maddie's condition has improved in previously implausible leaps and bounds since she began ingesting it early in 2014.

NO END IN SIGHT

Liz says it was "earth shattering" when Maddie was diagnosed with infant leukemia at 11 months old. The poor-prognosis cancer is rare, with a

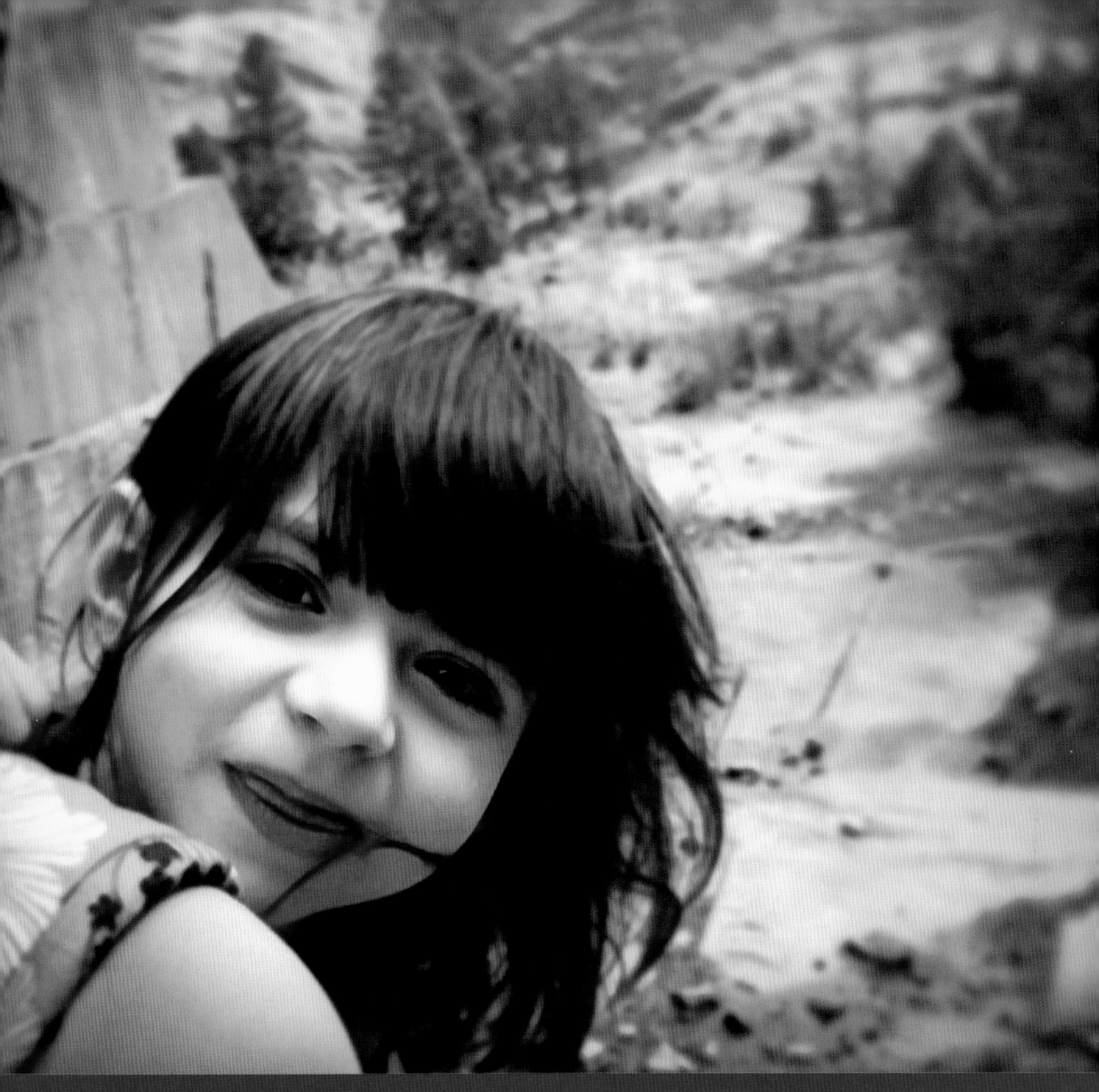

"WHEN YOU'RE WITH A GROUP OF PARENTS WHO HAVE ALL MADE THE CHOICE TO UPROOT THEIR LIVES—SOME ALL TOGETHER, SOME LIKE ME WHERE THE FAMILY IS SPLIT—YOU REALIZE THERE IS A LOT OF GOOD IN THE WORLD AND THERE ARE A LOT OF AMAZING PARENTS OUT THERE TRYING TO DO THE BEST FOR THEIR KIDS." —LIZ GORMAN

survival rate of just 50 percent, according to the Children's Cancer Research Fund. This kicked off a period of aggressive chemotherapy, which came to a halt when Maddie began having seizures as a 2-year-old. After each type of chemo she was receiving was eliminated as a potential cause for the seizures, Maddie was diagnosed with infantile spasms, a type of epilepsy that can cause severe developmental delays.

"If you get control quickly, you can mitigate those effects," Liz explains. "The longer this pattern of brain waves goes on, the worse the outcome. We quit chemo altogether and decided to call cancer the back-burner diagnosis."

Luckily, Maddie went into remission for leukemia and has, so far, gone without relapse. "I'm going to knock on some wood right now," Liz says, adding, "We still monitor everything very closely."

Epilepsy, however, was just beginning its cruel reign at the time she stopped chemo treatments. Maddie developed normally until its onset, and then did not. (Now 8, she functions like a 2-year-old. "But a pretty crazy 2-year-old," her mom adds lovingly). In the first year, the Gormans, living in North Carolina at the time, exhausted all of the first- and second-tier treatments for Maddie's type of epilepsy. They hung on through the torrent of ultimately unhelpful and dizzying assortments of drug cocktails. It was a "seesawing" of different combinations and dosages that interact with one another, spawning such a complex web of side effects that they couldn't be picked apart and traced back to their source.

When Maddie was 5, genetic testing revealed that she has a genetic abnormality called POLG, which means she is neurologically more sensitive to liver-toxic drugs, which many pharmaceuticals are. This limited the already shrinking pool of prescriptions Maddie had left to try. By then, her condition had evolved into a catastrophic type of epilepsy known as Lennox Gastaut Syndrome.

"At the time, she had just failed a medication that actually gave her some seizure freedom for a couple of months, so I was devastated," Liz says, remembering it as the only time her seemingly unbreakable hope faltered. "She had two months of being seizure-free and then they came back. During those two months I had just started running half-marathons. I thought maybe our battle was over. I didn't think things were going to be instantly better—I knew she was always going to be behind and that we had a ton of work to do—but I got those two months of time where … " She breaks off, collecting herself. " … where I thought we beat this stuff and could get to the period of healing," she continues. "Then, when they came back, they came back with a vengeance. They got bad quickly. They came back two days before Christmas."

Maddie was having nearly 500 seizures a day in clusters of 50 or 80 at a time, and spent 75 to 80 percent of her waking life seizing. Her most common type were myoclonics, a seizure defined by brief jerking of the muscles. She was also having three to five big tonic seizures, characterized by stiffening of the muscles, each day, as well as atonics, a dangerous type in which the muscles lose tone and Maddie would fall to the floor.

"She'd wake up, have a cluster of little head drops for 30 minutes, then some clarity during breakfast, then she'd have the head drops again, cluster with those, then she'd have a big seizure, then take a nap, wake up, and we'd do the same thing over and over," Liz says. "We were lucky if we got 15-minute windows to play and make the best of life."

Liz's certainty that a cure was around the corner was slipping, but she still believed it was possible to manage Maddie's epilepsy, and the option the family arrived at, having exhausted all of the others (they had even gone back and given things another try), was corpus callosotomy brain surgery, which she underwent at the age of 6 in July 2013.

The operation severed the corpus callosum, a thick connective tissue that connects the hemispheres of the brain, to interrupt the transmission of seizure signals from one side of the brain to the other and thereby stop Maddie's perilous atonic seizures.

And they did stop—for a teasingly encouraging three months. Then, on Thanksgiving Day, they returned. Two days later, on Maddie's 7th birthday, another seizure type that had ebbed resurfaced.

COLORADO BOUND

It was that day, Nov. 30, 2013, that the Gormans decided to move to Colorado.

Liz had heard of what was happening with cannabis to treat epilepsy via the Internet, but she was "so conservative that I went with brain surgery instead of that."

She found it hard to believe that there could be such an effective treatment for epilepsy that no one took seriously—a notion reinforced by Maddie's doctors, who pooh-poohed the idea. "I brought it up to them," she says, "and they all said 'Oh Liz, that's just silly, people always want to look for a more natural method

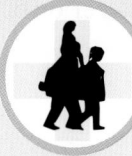

MEDICAL REFUGEE: Medical refugees are individuals or families who need medical cannabis to treat an illness but live in a state where it is still illegal. Families with children who suffer from epilepsy, in particular, relocate to Colorado or other states where medical marijuana is legal, so they can access the medicine without risking jail time or having their children taken away by state authorities. There is no exact count on the number of families who have moved as medical refugees to Colorado or other states, but news stories on CNN and in the *Chicago Tribune* have estimated that the number is in the hundreds. According to the Realm of Caring, the producers of Charlotte's Web CBD oil, the group has filled orders for more than 12,000 families.

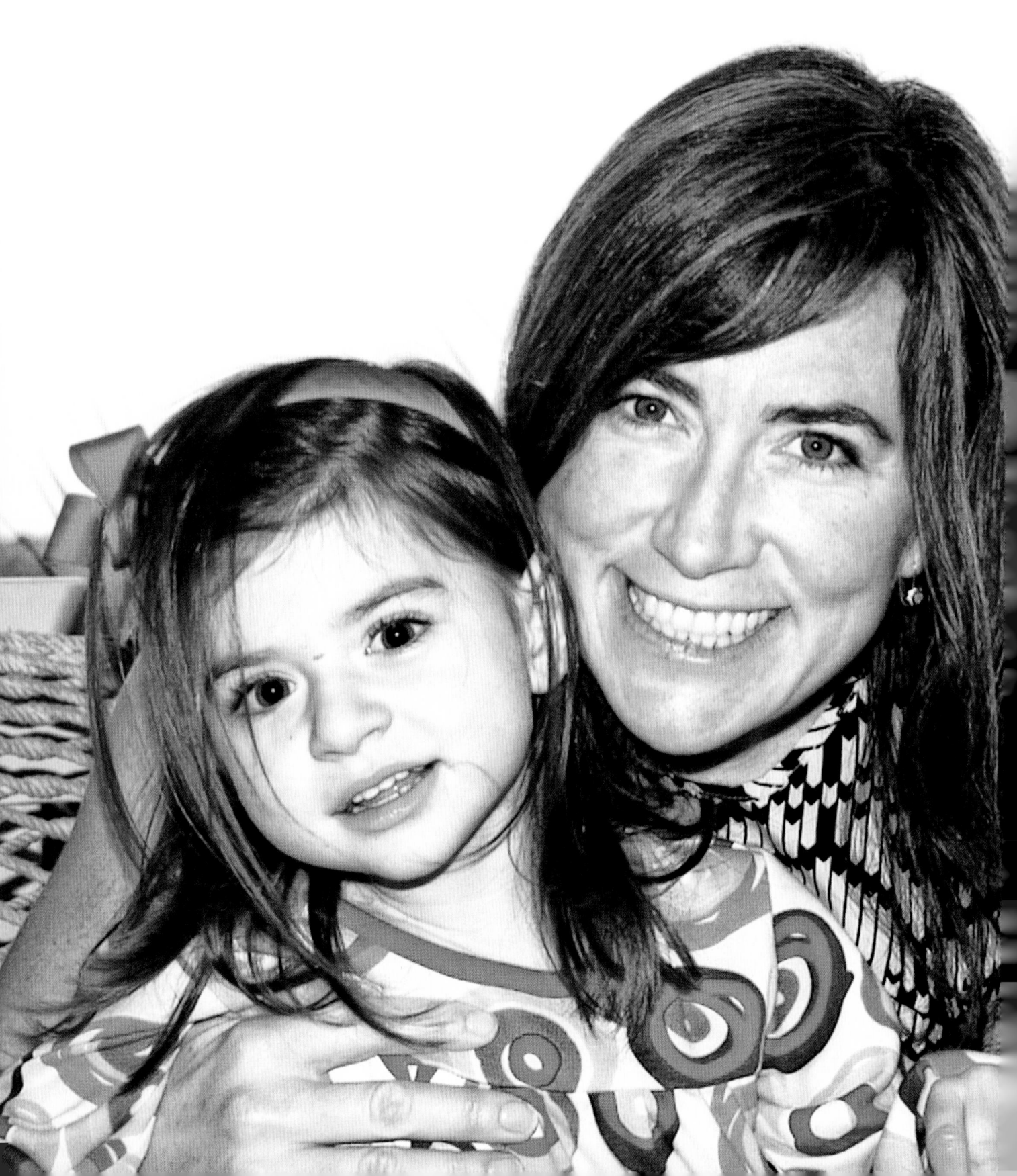

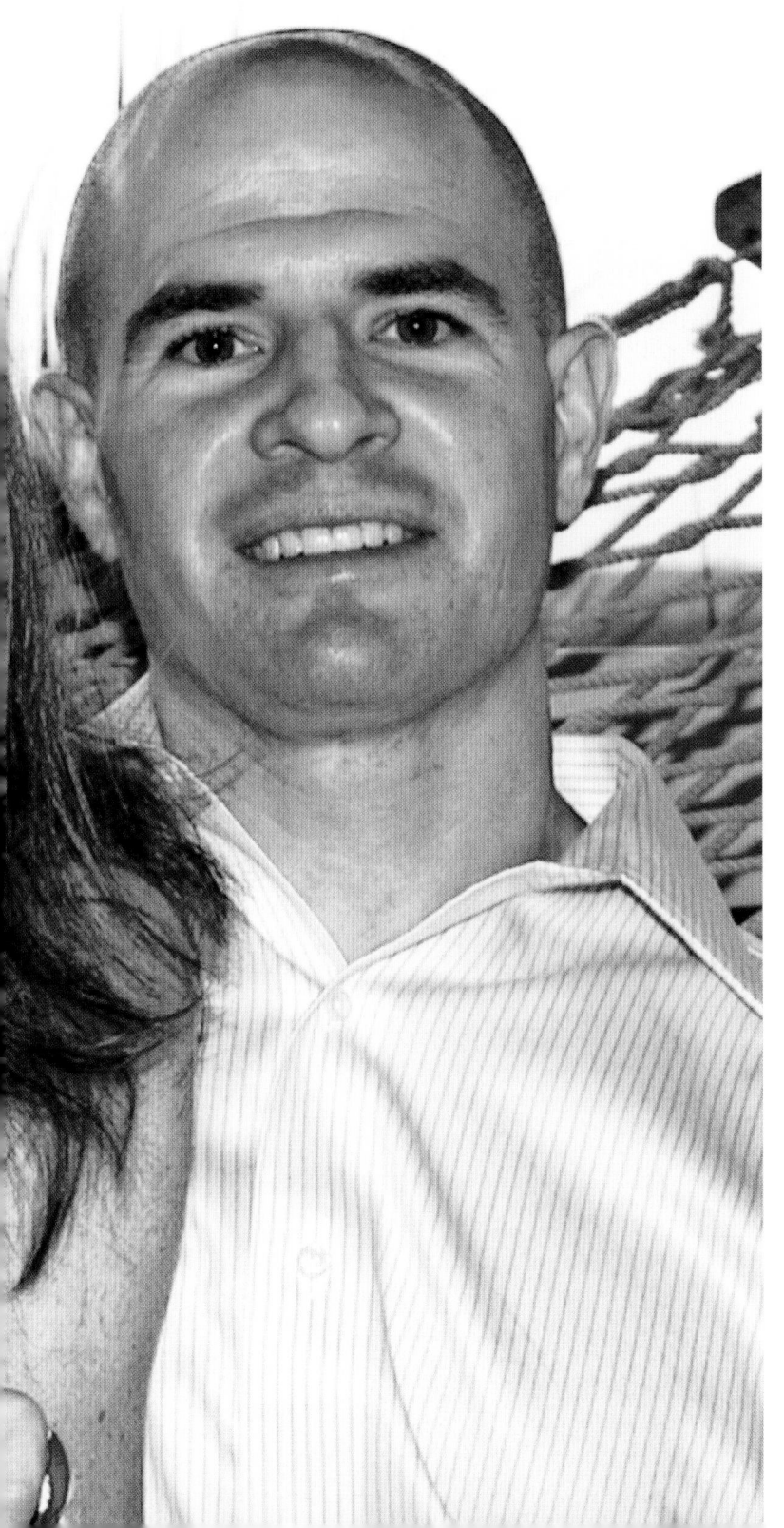

but don't you think if it helped seizures we'd know about it?'"

Still, with hope wearing thin, she added cannabis to the list of eleventh-hour efforts. And, just in case, she visited Colorado that October, when Maddie was still nearly seizure-free post-surgery, to find doctors and get on the waiting list for Charlotte's Web.

Just as Maddie's seizures made their unwelcomed return, the family received an email saying they were off the waiting list and able to order the medicine.

"SHE'D WAKE UP, HAVE A CLUSTER OF LITTLE HEAD DROPS FOR 30 MINUTES, THEN SOME CLARITY DURING BREAKFAST, THEN SHE'D HAVE THE HEAD DROPS AGAIN, CLUSTER WITH THOSE, THEN SHE'D HAVE A BIG SEIZURE, THEN TAKE A NAP, WAKE UP, AND WE'D DO THE SAME THING OVER AND OVER."

Liz and Maddie, accompanied by Liz's mother, were on a plane by Dec. 19. Her husband, Brandon Gorman, drove out with the bare necessities, including Maddie's seizure bed and equipment. A whirlwind house hunt later, they moved into a condo on Dec. 23. An infantry officer in the military, Brandon stayed through Christmas and then returned to North Carolina, where he was stationed at the time. (He's now in Rhode Island.)

Before relocating to Colorado in pursuit of Charlotte's Web, Liz, as positive as she is, was conditioned by years of unsuccessful treatments to expect a letdown. She signed just a six-month lease upon arrival, sure that cannabis would soon be just another flopped solution to cross off the dwindling list of last resorts.

Following brain surgery, Maddie was down to 100 seizures a day when the mother-daughter duo settled into their new home. Five days into the Charlotte's Web treatment, long-lost motor skills resurfaced. After two weeks, her seizures were down 50 percent. At the six-month mark, with 80 to 90 percent reduction in seizures, Liz finally realized that this experiment just might be working.

OFF THE PHARMACEUTICALS

Today, Maddie's seizures still crop up, although far less often, and for a fraction of the duration. When we speak, Liz is weaning Maddie off of one of her two last pharmaceuticals, and considering doing the same with the other down the line.

Through it all, Liz has been by Maddie's side. Or, rather, just behind her, ready to catch her if she falls—literally. Before Maddie's leukemia diagnosis, Liz sold real estate, and before that she worked with children with severe autism—experience that came in handy in raising Maddie. Once the epilepsy began, Liz's full-time job became keeping Maddie safe, and she had her work cut out for her when the little girl was suffering hundreds of seizures a day. Although Maddie is able to walk, drop seizures can strike at any moment, bringing her crashing to the ground. Rather than confine Maddie to a wheelchair or equip her with a helmet, Liz opts to walk a foot or two behind her, clutching the leash of a harness, ready to catch her when they do.

But that leash is slackening as Maddie improves. The development that froze when Maddie started having seizures has jumpstarted, aided by ABA, or Applied Behavior Analysis, a therapy mostly used to help children with autism. Maddie now knows the ABCs, colors, and numbers, and, as of this writing, was working on recognizing words. "We're gonna teach this kid to read!" Liz exclaims, with a touch of lingering disbelief.

"She's so much more alert, aware, and interactive with the world," she says, noting that they hope to have Maddie in school by the fall. "These things were out of the realm of possibility before we got here."

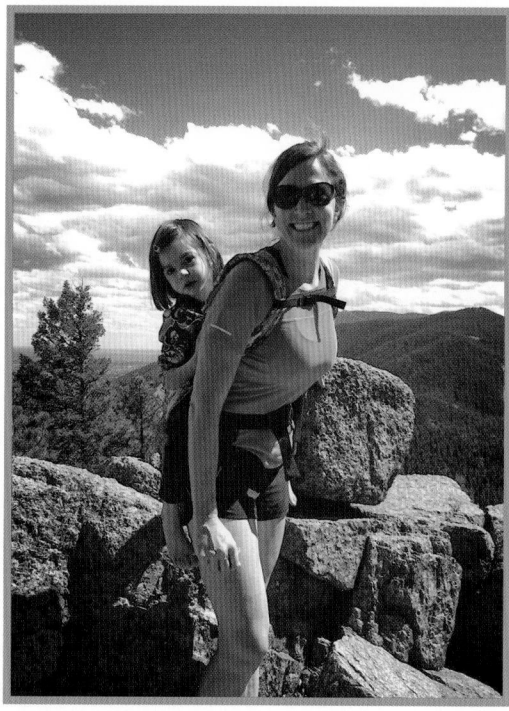

These once-impossible things have Liz savoring the first taste of her own life in seven years. Unheard of in the pre-Charlotte's Web days, Liz can leave Maddie with a babysitter, a luxury she's been utilizing to go rock climbing with friends. She recently left her mother in charge for two days while in Washington, D.C., to lobby for HR 1653, the Charlotte's Web Medical Access Act, which was introduced in the spring of 2015 and, if passed, would exclude CBD treatments from the federal definition of marijuana.

But, while Liz and "monkey" (or "booger bear," or any other of the terms of endearment she showers on Maddie) are making the best of it in Colorado, it's not easy living apart from her husband and her family.

"Our family has lived apart for a year and a half now in order to have access to this medicine," she says, touching on the bittersweet reality many medical refugee families face. The Gormans are just one of estimated hundreds of similar families who have fled to Colorado to obtain cannabis medicine for their children, and have clustered around Colorado Springs, where Charlotte's Web is distributed. Liz and Maddie find comfort in this community.

"It's great being among a group of people who have all been through as much as we have," Liz says. "When you're with a group of parents who have all made the choice to uproot their lives—some all together, some like me where the family is split—you realize there is a lot of good in the world and there are a lot of amazing parents out there trying to do the best for their kids."

As for Maddie, the little girl is now freer than ever from the prison of her condition, and, based on Liz's description, she has a sunny personality to rival her mom's. She's lovable, sweet, bubbly, and is known to get Liz's attention by pulling her head around for a kiss. Things are finally looking as bright for the Gormans as Liz always held out hope that they would.

"I am getting to watch little miracles happen around me all the time," she says. "It's a pretty cool thing to be a part of."

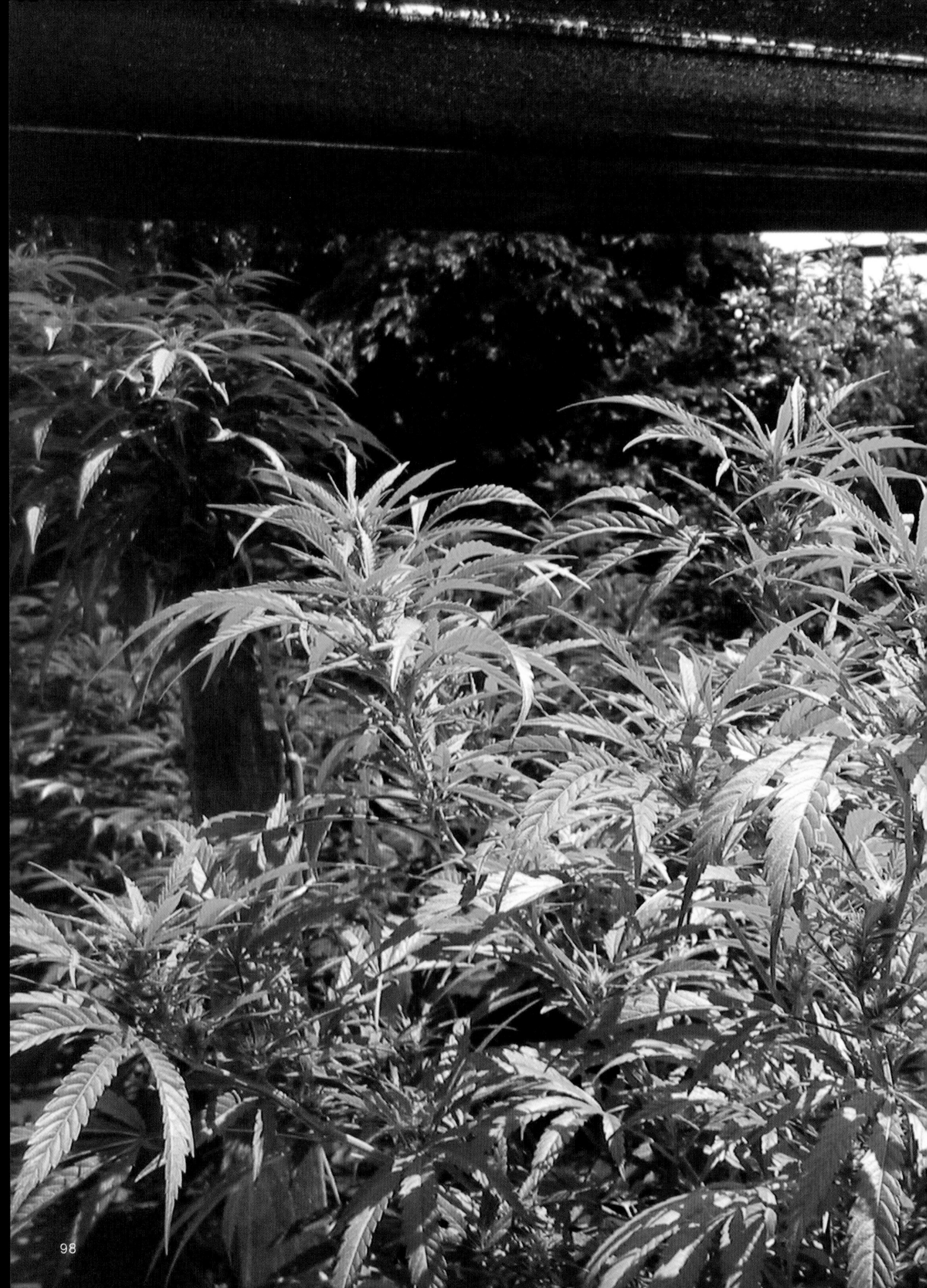

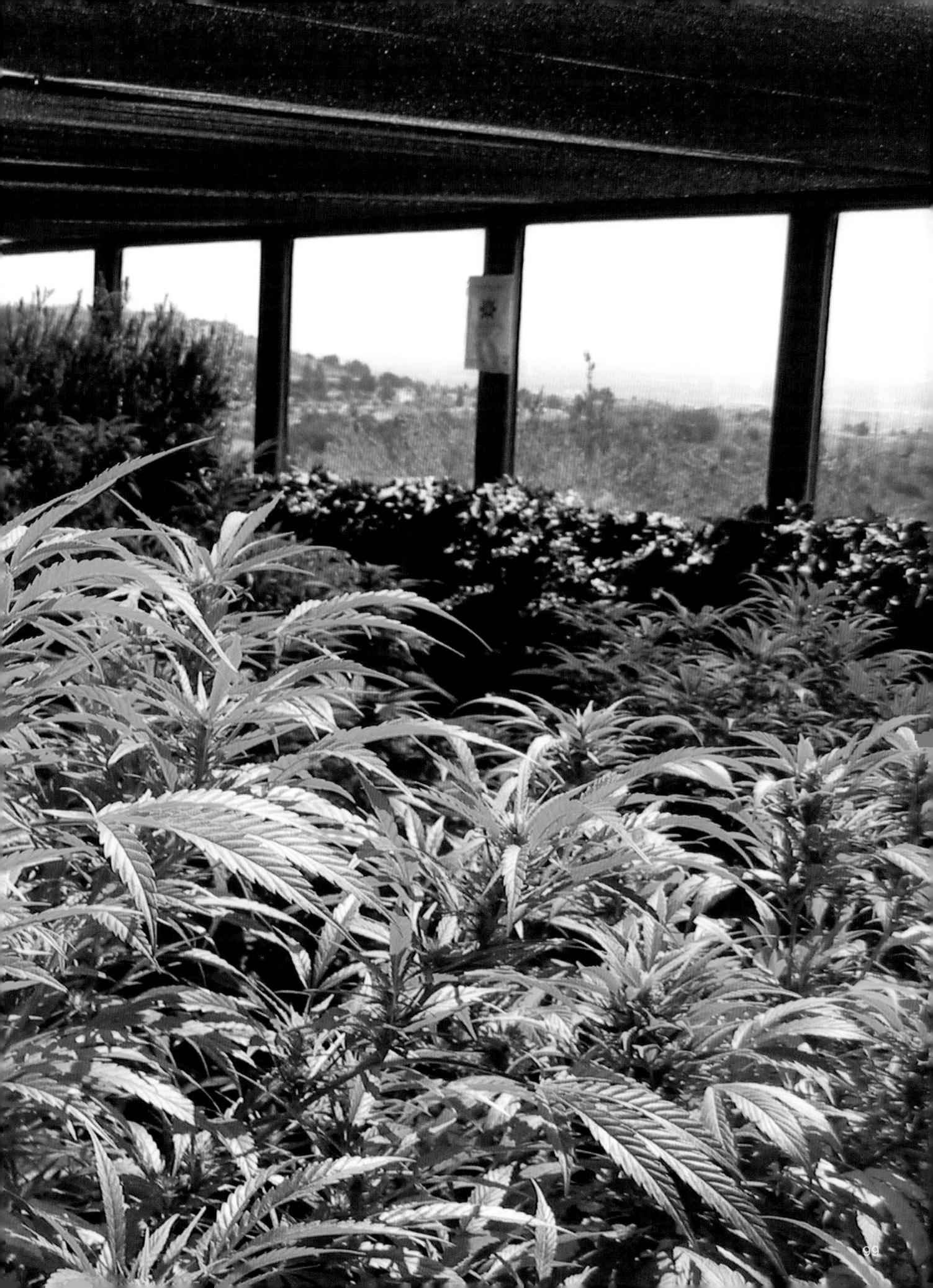

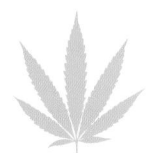

MARK DIPASQUALE

Age 39 / **PTSD** / Rochester, New York

During his two tours of Iraq, between 2005 and 2007, Mark DiPasquale served as a door gunner aboard a UH-1N. He describes the aircraft as "an air assault attack platform that was used for a lot of convoys, protection [tasks], raids—anything they would use a helicopter for, from surveillance to reconnaissance to shooting somebody."

He returned for his second tour despite having sustained an injury during a hard-landing crash in 2005 that resulted in severe migraines. In addition to the headaches, he had sleeping problems and emerging PTSD, and became hooked on pain and sleeping pills.

"It's part of the American and military culture to take over-the-counter and prescribed drugs," he says, noting their ubiquity among his fellow service members.

Indeed, seven out of 10 Americans take a prescription drug, more than half take two, and 20 percent are on five or more, according to a 2013 study by the Mayo Clinic. Following antibiotics, anti-depressants and opioids are the most commonly prescribed medications. As a concentrated version of greater American culture (or, as Mark puts it, "the core of this American apple pie image"), the military is also wrought with prescription drug use. Pentagon data shows that the number of pain medication prescriptions written by military doctors spiked from nearly 867,000 in 2001 to 3.8 million in 2009.

Because of what he now believes was a combination of his previous injury, high stress, and sleeping pills, Mark had to be medevac'd back to base during a mission in 2006 because of panic symptoms and heart palpitations. He was temporarily retired from the military because of migraines and PTSD in 2008, after 13 years of active duty, and officially medically retired in 2010. He took a job doing security for a private contractor in Iraq for three years. "It didn't help my PTSD," Mark says, "it added to it."

The VA's answer to his issues was a laundry list of prescriptions—anywhere from 10 to 12 different medications taken each day. "They really hop you up," notes Mark, who was granted 100-percent level disability by the VA in 2014.

Around 2010, Mark realized he wanted to live a healthier life, and by 2012 he was off of all over-the-counter and doctor-prescribed medications, using just cannabis to treat his symptoms. "With an anxiety disorder, like PTSD, it has helped with all of my issues, as far as sleeping, anxiety, stress, and anger levels," he says. "It doesn't make me perfect, but it manages the symptoms."

New York, where Mark lives with his wife and three children, recently passed a medical marijuana law, and he is looking forward to legally purchasing cannabis from dispensaries in his area. Vaporizing whole plant cannabis is just one way he keeps healthy, along with a vegan diet and active lifestyle. And this boosted, vigorous take on life is what he would describe as being "high"—a word he doesn't eschew when it comes to discuss-

ing cannabis. The high, he says, is part of the plant's medicinal value.

"I actually *am* using it to get high," he says. "This is what I've learned through my studies: People have demonized the word 'high,' when being high is healthy. Being low is not. Being down, depressed—that isn't good. By 'high,' it means I'm getting happy and healthy. It means that I'm about to go on a run for four miles, and come back and eat fruits and vegetables. It's a healthy attitude."

He's just as passionate about hemp, a cannabis variety that, while often confused with marijuana, is not psychoactive and is cultivated for its broad range of industrial purposes. Hemp seeds, to name one of these uses, pack a potent nutritional punch—they are high in protein, omega fatty acids, fiber, antioxidants and minerals. With this in mind, Mark recently helped form an organization that targets malnutrition and hunger by replacing rice production in the small West African country of Gambia with hemp. (Visit facebook.com/Hemp4the-HomelessofGambia for more information).

Stateside, he is inspiring other veterans to consider cannabis as part of a holistic approach to healing through his work with the Veterans Cannabis Collective, a volunteer-run group he co-founded in 2014.

He comes up against a lot of fear and misunderstanding among veterans with whom he speaks, and hopes to disrupt that old way of thinking—the blind alle-

SEVEN OUT OF 10 AMERICANS TAKE A PRESCRIPTION DRUG, MORE THAN HALF TAKE TWO, AND 20 PERCENT ARE ON FIVE OR MORE, ACCORDING TO A 2013 STUDY BY THE MAYO CLINIC.

giance to unhealthy habits that are engrained in American and military culture and, he adds, spurred by prescription-pad-wielding doctors.

"If [veterans] are so concerned about the bad, negative image of cannabis, I'd like to encourage them to take a look at what kind of food we're eating—these are the same people eating double cheeseburgers and drinking pop all day," he says. "I'll talk to someone and think, 'You're telling me you just came back from the bar, took a couple of Percocet, and are about to eat a cheeseburger—and you're concerned about consuming a flower?'"

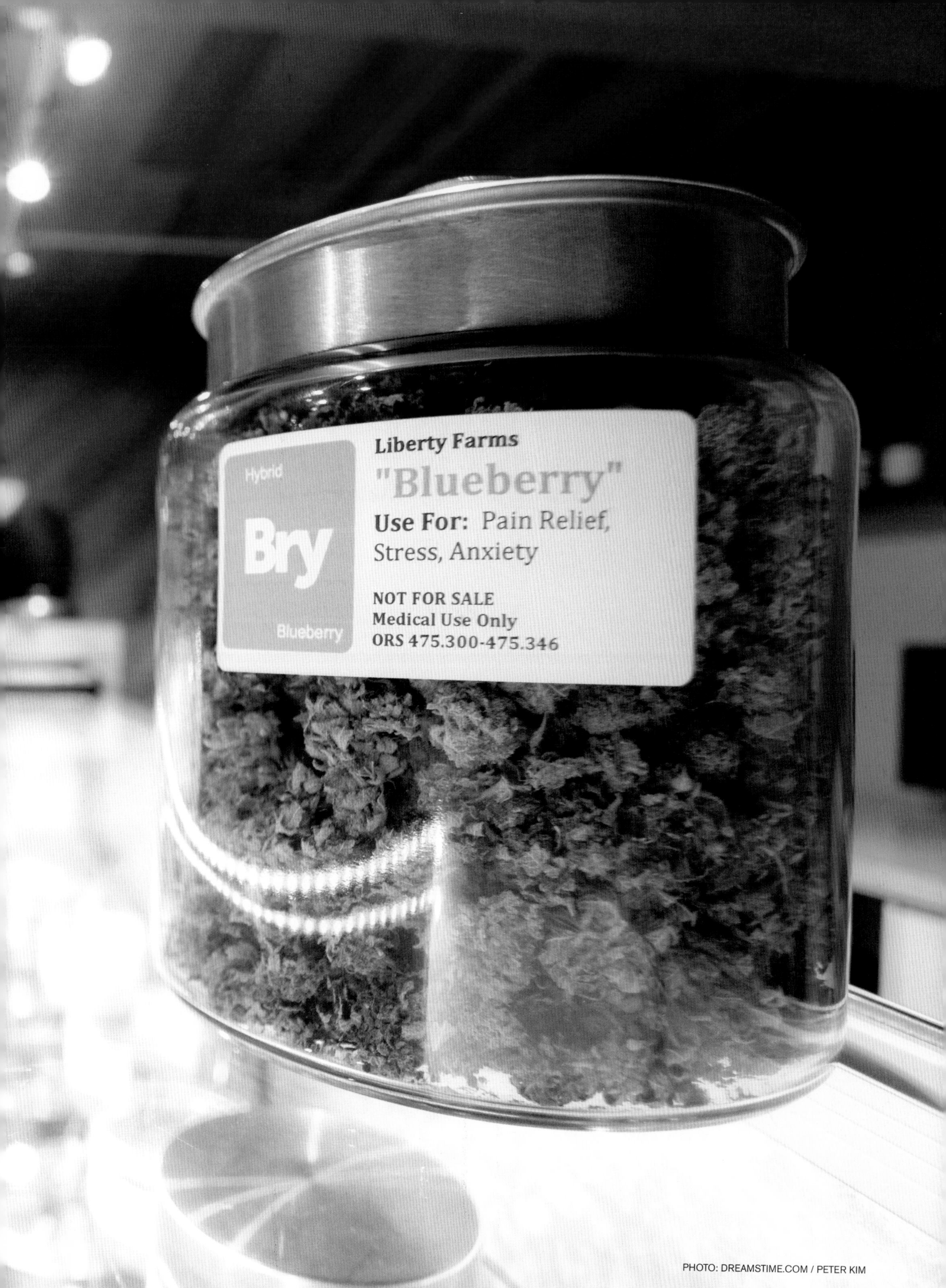

Liberty Farms
"Blueberry"
Use For: Pain Relief, Stress, Anxiety
NOT FOR SALE
Medical Use Only
ORS 475.300-475.346
Hybrid
Bry
Blueberry

PHOTO: DREAMSTIME.COM / PETER KIM

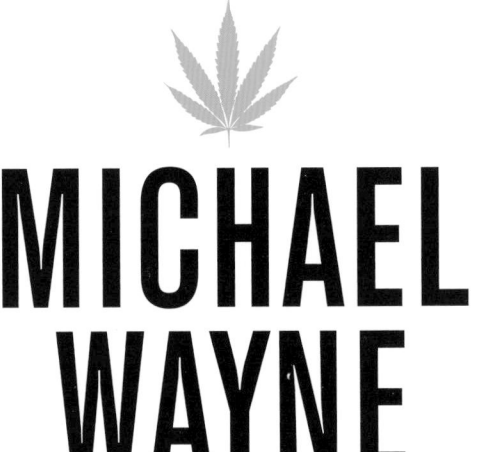

MICHAEL WAYNE

Age 62 / **AIDS** / Gibsonton, Florida

By the time doctors realized Michael Wayne had AIDS, in 2004, they said the disease had to have been progressing, unsuspectingly, for 10 to 15 years.

Michael lived in Tampa, Florida, at the time, where he was studying Traditional Chinese Medicine (TCM), a several-thousand-year-old Chinese tradition of healing practices that include herbs and acupuncture.

"I had very abundant health from practicing different martial arts and healing arts, so I probably fared better than your normal Joe who gets the disease, and that may be why I was able to sustain myself for so long while this was eating away at me," Michael says.

Underneath the surface, however, his immune system was disintegrating. He came down with shingles in 2004, causing severe nerve damage in his back. The shingles led doctors to discover that Michael had an astonishingly low T cell count—a type of white blood cell that is needed for cell-mediated immunity—and diagnose him with AIDS.

"I almost died," he says. "They didn't know if I would make it or not."

Around this time, he moved from Tampa to Gibsonton, where he has lived since, and began highly active antiretroviral therapy, or HAART, which uses a team of drugs to attack different viral points and reduce the overall impact of HIV/AIDS on the body. "I'm on my fourth set of those," Michael says. "You'll take it for a while and it either works or it doesn't. They only have so many in the medicine cabinet, so when you run out, that's the end of the road."

"IF YOU CAN BE HAPPY, MAINTAIN YOUR APPETITE, SUPPRESS YOUR NAUSEA, AND YOU'RE NOT DOING ANYTHING TOXIC TO YOUR BODY, WHAT CAN BE BETTER?"

The shingles episode resulted in neuropathic pain, for which Michael was previously taking a host of prescriptions—"morphine sulfates, Percocet, hydrocodone, you name it, at one time or another I've tried it in different combinations."

About three years ago, he became fed up with the "mental fog" he lived in and the harsh side effects, including nausea, and decided to try using cannabis. He discovered that it reduced his queasiness and neuropathic pain, made antidepressants no longer necessary, and helped him lower the number of narcotics and other medications he takes. He began growing it in his backyard and juicing the raw plants, to be drank like other juiced fruits and vegetables.

"For absolute certainty there are benefits in cannabis, and they are varied and profound, and there is a definite place for it in medicine," Michael says. "If you can be happy, maintain your appetite, suppress your nausea, and you're not doing anything toxic to your body, what can be better? How many medicines do you know of that can treat as many things as cannabis? None. There is nothing to compare it to."

He says that the single most important role cannabis plays in his life is to support his current HAART treatment. "It helps me be more compliant in taking my medicine. If you're calm and not being affected, and don't have the mind fog and can control your sleep patterns, it's easier to take your pills. And at this point, if I lose another regimen, they may have another for me to try, they may not."

Before trying cannabis, Michael didn't often go out in public—he was too nervous about contracting illnesses because of his compromised immune system. To the amazement of his doctors, his T cells have skyrocketed "to the point where you can't tell my counts from a normal person's," Michael says. Between his Chinese medicine, martial arts, and cannabis, his quality of life has been bolstered to the point where he is not just getting out of the house, but he's actively giving back to others. He became an ordained Christian minister in 2006, and has since been doing outreach to homeless veterans, and gathering and distributing health, hygiene and food supplies to the homeless in his area.

For Michael Wayne, it can't get much better than giving back to the community.

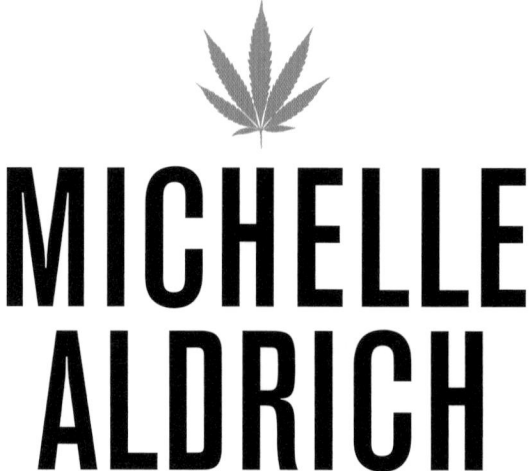

MICHELLE ALDRICH

Age 68 / **Cancer** / San Francisco

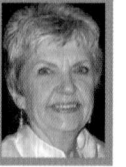

Growing up, Michelle Aldrich learned about the world and its far-flung destinations from postcards that her father sent while traveling as an airline pilot. With the arrival of each new note, Michelle and her mother would crack open the atlas and pinpoint her father's latest whereabouts on a map.

As a result, Michelle, who has lived in San Francisco for 40 years with her husband, Michael Aldrich, nurses a healthy case of wanderlust. A recent battle with lung cancer only spurred her desire for globetrotting adventures. "My bucket list is to travel the world," she says.

Doctors discovered a cancerous tumor on Michelle's right lung in January 2012, when she was 65 years old. As a marijuana legalization activist with decades of advo-cacy under her belt—she and Michael met at The First People's Pot Conference in Washington, D.C., in the early '70s—Michelle didn't hesitate to consider cannabis as part of her treatment. Upon diagnosis, she turned to her already robust medical cannabis network for help.

The Wo/Men's Alliance for Medical Marijuana (WAMM), a patient collective about an hour and a half south in Santa Cruz, provided her with a cancer-targeting whole cannabis plant extract called Milagro Oil. From a cannabis author and chef, she received guidance on diet, and began avoiding sugar, wheat, dairy, red meat and processed foods. Another doctor in her circle advised her to take various supplements, including omega fish oil and vitamin D.

Michelle waited to use the cannabis oil until the location and size of the cancer was confirmed. After several tests, it was determined to be Stage 3A poorly differentiated non-small cell metastatic adenocarcinoma. Bulky, cancerous lymph nodes were standing in the way of operating on the tumor, and Michelle was put on a chemotherapy treatment to shrink them. Springtime unfolded with chemotherapy sessions and 72 days of ingesting Milagro Oil. Unsure what the outcome would be, Michelle drew up a will and prepared for the worst.

In April, a CT scan showed dramatically reduced lymph nodes and a tumor half the size it had previously been. She finished her round of Milagro Oil on May 16 and had surgery May 18, when six lymph nodes and the shrunken remains of her tumor were removed. Her doctors didn't expect the chemo to have such a thorough effect, and in just a matter of months. Michelle, who was upfront with them about her cannabis use, believes the oil played a critical role in her recovery.

"My cancer was healed by a combination of Milagro Oil, chemotherapy, healthy diet, acupuncture, brilliant, empathetic doctors, and loving support from many friends," Michelle is quoted as saying in the online medical cannabis journal *O'Shaughnessy's* (beyondthc. com). "I truly believe that if it wasn't for the oil I would not be alive today."

She remains cancer-free, and continues to use the oil every night—a dose the size of a grain of rice—as a preventative measure. And she has not taken her renewed health for granted. Since her recovery, she and Michael set sail for Hawaii and Europe on cruises, and, as of this writing, had two more cruises on the horizon—a seven-day voyage along the California coast, and another to Alaska.

While hopscotching across Europe for the first time during a cruise in 2014, Michelle climbed to the top of the Parthenon in Athens, saw the Vatican in Rome, and beheld the famous "Blue Mosque" in Istanbul. And, of course, she paid homage at the Hash Marihuana & Hemp Museum in Barcelona.

CANCER & CANNABIS: Cancer is caused when abnormal cells in the human body multiply uncontrollably, resulting in tumors that can rapidly spread to other parts of the body and ultimately kill the patient. Medical marijuana has long been used to reduce nausea and promote appetite in people undergoing cancer treatment, but recent research shows that cannabis can also be useful for treating the cancer itself. A study published in 2014 showed that THC can cause cancer cells in mice to self-destruct, and can slow down the advance of brain and breast cancer. Other preliminary research and anecdotal reports suggest that cannabis is also useful against colorectal cancer, skin cancer and prostate cancer.

Researchers suspect that marijuana exhibits these cancer-fighting properties because it stimulates the body's endocannabinoid system, which, among other functions, controls the recycling of cell materials, an essential component of anti-tumor responses. *Sources: American Cancer Society, Leafscience.com, NORML.*

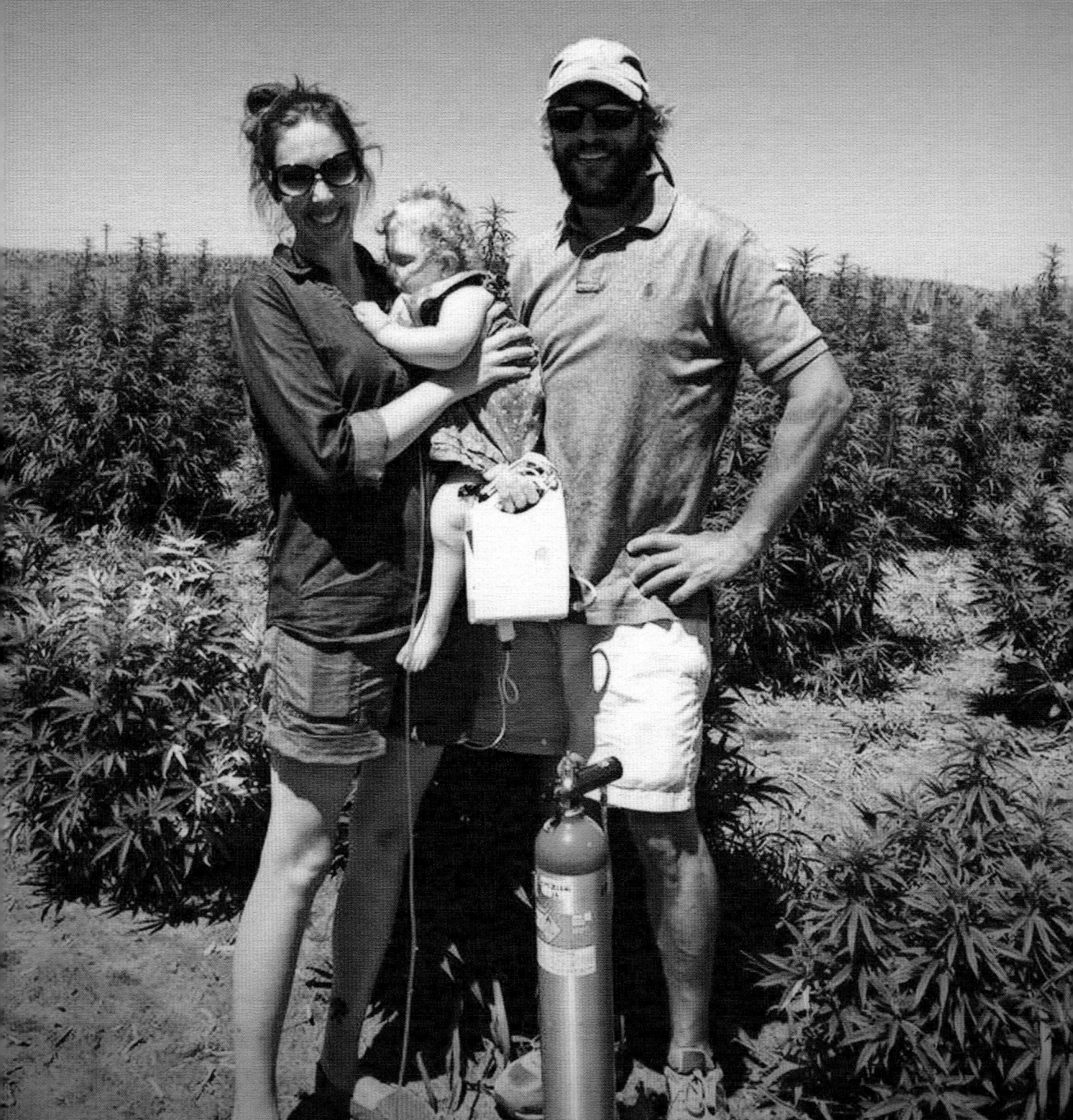

"HOPE HAS A WAY."

—NICOLE MATTISON

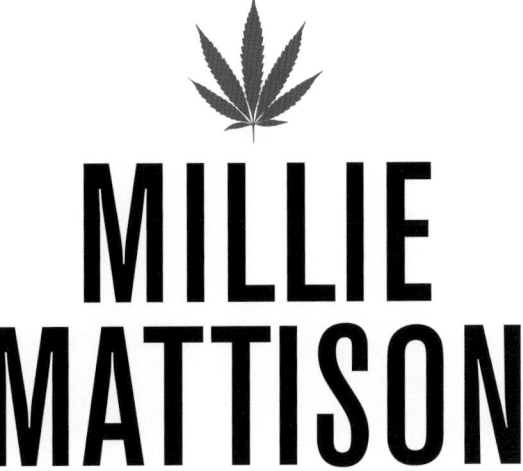

MILLIE MATTISON

Age 3 / **Infantile Spasms** / Colorado Springs, Colorado

Nicole Mattison remembers the call well. It was the summer of 2012, and she was at the radio station, an NPR affiliate in Nashville, where she managed corporate supporters. She was attempting to return to a normal routine after a traumatic development in her family the week before, when her 3-month-old daughter Millie was diagnosed with a type of seizures known as Infantile Spasms (IS).

The possibility of normalcy disappeared, however, when her husband Penn called from the hospital where Millie was being treated. "He was just frantic," Nicole says. "He said that the neurologist said she was going to be severely retarded and had a slim survival rate." Nicole rushed to the hospital to hear the ominous news in person.

IS, which typically surfaces between 4 and 8 months old, has a high risk of developmental delay. In a 2006 paper published by the American Epilepsy Society titled "Infantile Spasms: Little Seizures, BIG Consequences," author W. Donald Shields, MD, calls it "arguably the most interesting, but also the most enigmatic, of all the epilepsy syndromes." While the frequency of spasms often decreases by mid-childhood, more than half of children with IS will go on to have other types of seizures, according to the National Institute of Neurological Disorders and Stroke. It's imperative to manage them as soon as possible to preserve the child's potential for normal cognitive development.

"The prognosis, even now, is very grim for Infantile Spasms if you can't get them under control," Nicole says. Millie started medications and the Ketogenic Diet, a high-fat, low-carbohydrate food regimen that targets hard-to-control types of epilepsy, and spent the summer in and out of the hospital. With no luck controlling the seizures, Millie was experiencing "failure to thrive," a condition in which babies are not gaining weight at a necessary rate. She was fed through a tube, and struggled with gastroesophageal reflux disease (GERD). Nicole quit her job in August, around the time Millie came down with pneumonia. That fall, having been told by Millie's existing doctors that they had done all they could, the family took Millie to the Cincinnati Children's Hospital.

"We were happy that we at least had her and were able to love her," Nicole says. "But we were grieving her infancy. Neither one of our other children were special needs, so we were shoved into a world that we knew nothing about."

Just as they began to adjust, Millie's dosages of Sabril, an anticonvulsant used to treat seizures and infantile spasm, were increased. "And that's when she went to sleep," Nicole says. "She slept for 23 to 24 hours a day. She wasn't progressing. She was still having seizures. And they kept increasing the dosages."

Millie spent 2013 bedridden. That summer, severe acidosis—acid build-up in her body—had her in and out of the hospital. During one visit, "she just crashed," says Nicole. "Her kidneys were failing. She wasn't urinating. She had blood in her stomach and stool from a stomach bleed from the acidosis." At Nicole's request, Millie was switched to a natural version of the Ketogenic Diet, which it turned out had been aggravating her acidosis, and the 1-year-old finally began gaining weight.

THE CNN DOCUMENTARY

As this was unfolding, Penn saw *Weed*, a widely viewed and discussed CNN documentary about medical marijuana in which Dr. Sanjay Gupta famously reverses his stance from skeptic to believer. It shares the story of a little girl named Charlotte Figi, whose heartbreaking battle with Dravet Syndrome (a severe form of intractable epilepsy) gave her hundreds of seizures a week. These seizures were amazingly reduced when she began using cannabis. Charlotte's parents, having exhausted all treatment options, developed a cannabis oil that is high in CBD, which is non-psychoactive, and low in psychoactive THC. Her seizure frequency plummeted. Today known as Charlotte's Web, the cannabis oil is prominently known for its use to treat pediatric epilepsy.

The Mattisons were immediately intrigued upon hearing about Charlotte's Web on CNN. They dove into research and connected with other families dealing with pediatric epilepsy on the Internet. In October 2013, they asked Millie's neurologist in Cincinnati about it.

"She said, 'You know it's illegal here, so I can't recommend it, but I do recommend you do what you can to help Millie,'" Nicole recounts. "On the drive from Cincinnati to Nashville, we were booking our flights to Colorado, making an appointment with [a doctor], and learning what we needed to do to get a legal marijuana card there." They decided that instead of splitting up, like many medical marijuana refugee families do, the whole family would relocate and start over in Colorado.

"We said, 'For us it's all or nothing. We're all gonna go for Millie,'" Nicole says. "We sold my husband's landscape business in the dead of winter, packed up what we could, donated the rest, and drove out in early January."

CHARLOTTE'S WEB

On March 6, 2014, Millie's 2nd birthday, the Mattisons received an email saying that their order for Charlotte's Web was ready to be picked up.

"I will never forget the first dose she took," Nicole says. "My family had been in town for her birthday and my husband left to take them to the airport. We'd given it

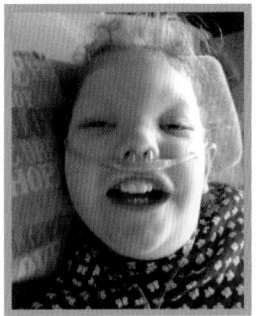

to her shortly before they left so they could say 'Oh yay!' The result was amazing. She was wide-awake. I was taking pictures and sending them, saying, 'I can't believe you're missing this, you left too soon!'"

The 2-year-old opened her eyes and looked around, absorbing the sights that surrounded her like she never had before. Eventually, she began making eye contact and developed more movement abilities. "She used to be floppy as a ragdoll, and now a year later she sits up on her own and holds her head up," Nicole says.

In October of that year, the little girl who once suffered hundreds of seizures a day went a miraculous 48 hours without a single one. Today, she's nearly down to zero. Nicole now works for the Realm of Caring Foundation, the Colorado nonprofit behind Charlotte's Web, and Penn is a stay-at-home dad.

Nicole is grateful that the family never gave in to the defeated prognosis proffered by Millie's doctors and Western medicine, generally. For her family, she says cannabis is proof that "hope has a way."

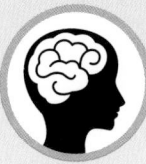

EPILEPSY: Epilepsy is a neurological disorder most commonly associated with seizures. Extreme cases can provoke hundreds of uncontrollable seizures per day. Studies and anecdotal evidence suggest that cannabis, and CBD oil in particular, can help control seizures in some cases where pharmaceutical interventions have failed to make an impact. The treatment has shown great promise in helping epileptic children live normal lives. *Sources: Epilepsy Foundation of Colorado, Realm of Caring Foundation. Illustration by Freepik.com*

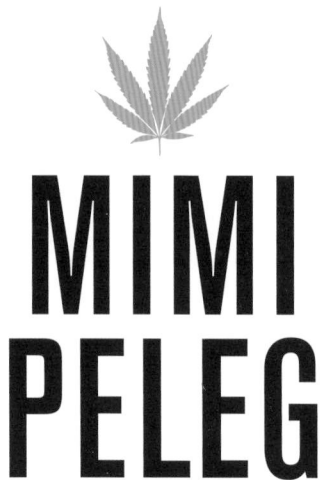

MIMI PELEG

Age 53 / **Endometrial Cancer, PTSD** / Bonny Doon, California

A medley of miscellaneous items communes in the center of Mimi Peleg's green-tiled kitchen table. Huddled among the salt and pepper shakers, a small plant potted in a coffee mug, and a cup of assorted pens are several mason jars containing various strains of cannabis. "Key Lime Pie" is written in Sharpie across the lid of one. Another is identified as "UK Cheese" on a strip of masking tape.

Mimi selects a jar and extracts a few clusters of olive-green buds, placing them in a grinder where they are milled into specks that, moments later, she rolls into a joint. She talks as her hands work, beginning with her time as a medical cannabis patient trainer in Israel. As I listen, I sip a creamy green smoothie that she handed me upon arrival—a nutritional powerhouse made with cashew milk, coconut yogurt, avocado, the juices of a host of vegetables gleaned from the local farmers market and raw, juiced cannabis plant. Around us, the spacious house is on its way to being set up. Mimi recently moved in to the home, a rental deep in the wooded periphery of Santa Cruz County, California, and her wife and son are soon to follow from Israel, where the family lived since 2009.

There, Mimi worked training new patients in the country's nascent government-run medical marijuana program. "I'd get them thinking about their priorities, explain a bit about how cannabis works, and then I would start to help them understand which method of using cannabis would best help them attain their goals," she says.

"WHILE I WAS IN THE HOSPITAL, THE CANNABIS HELPED GIVE ME AN APPETITE, GET ME TO SLEEP, AND KEEP ME OUT OF PAIN."

Mimi has used cannabis, herself, for many years and for varied reasons. She turned to it during her battle with endometrial cancer, which she was diagnosed with in late 2011, while living in Israel. Because of its medical legality there, Mimi was able to vaporize cannabis while recovering from a full hysterectomy in the hospital.

"While I was in the hospital, the cannabis helped give me an appetite, get me to sleep, and keep me out of pain," she says. "I wasn't in pain—and I'm a big ol' baby."

She refused radiation and chemotherapy, opting instead to proceed with intensive cannabis oil as her cancer treatment. It wasn't easy—heavy doses of the strong extract kept her groggy and lethargic throughout the treatment period—but it was effective. Just two weeks before my visit, a CT scan assured that she remains cancer free. To keep it that way, she uses a small dose of the oil each month.

But today, Mimi mostly uses cannabis to curb the PTSD she's incurred from a string of wounding experiences, including sexual abuse, her time as a soldier in the Israeli army, and the murder by terrorists

of her best friend. She first moved to Israel as a young adult with hopes of attending college through a scholarship available to citizens. But, she says with a deep-voiced chuckle, "I changed my citizenship, was rejected from college, and received my draft notice." She served in the Israeli army for three years before moving back to the United States, where she attended UC Berkeley.

Eventually settling in Santa Cruz, she met her wife, who is Israeli, on a trip to Israel a dozen years ago and it "was love at first sight," she says. Her own experience with PTSD led her to work for a period with the Santa Cruz-based organization Multidisciplinary Association for Psychedelic Studies (MAPS), as a clinical research associate for a study of MDMA-assisted psychotherapy for PTSD. The couple decided to move back to Israel in 2009 with their then-4-and-a-half-year-old son, but Mimi ultimately wearied of the war-torn environment and worried about the impact it was having on her son.

"My son is also dealing with a lot of PTSD" from living in Israel, she says, now roaming the property's rambling and fer-

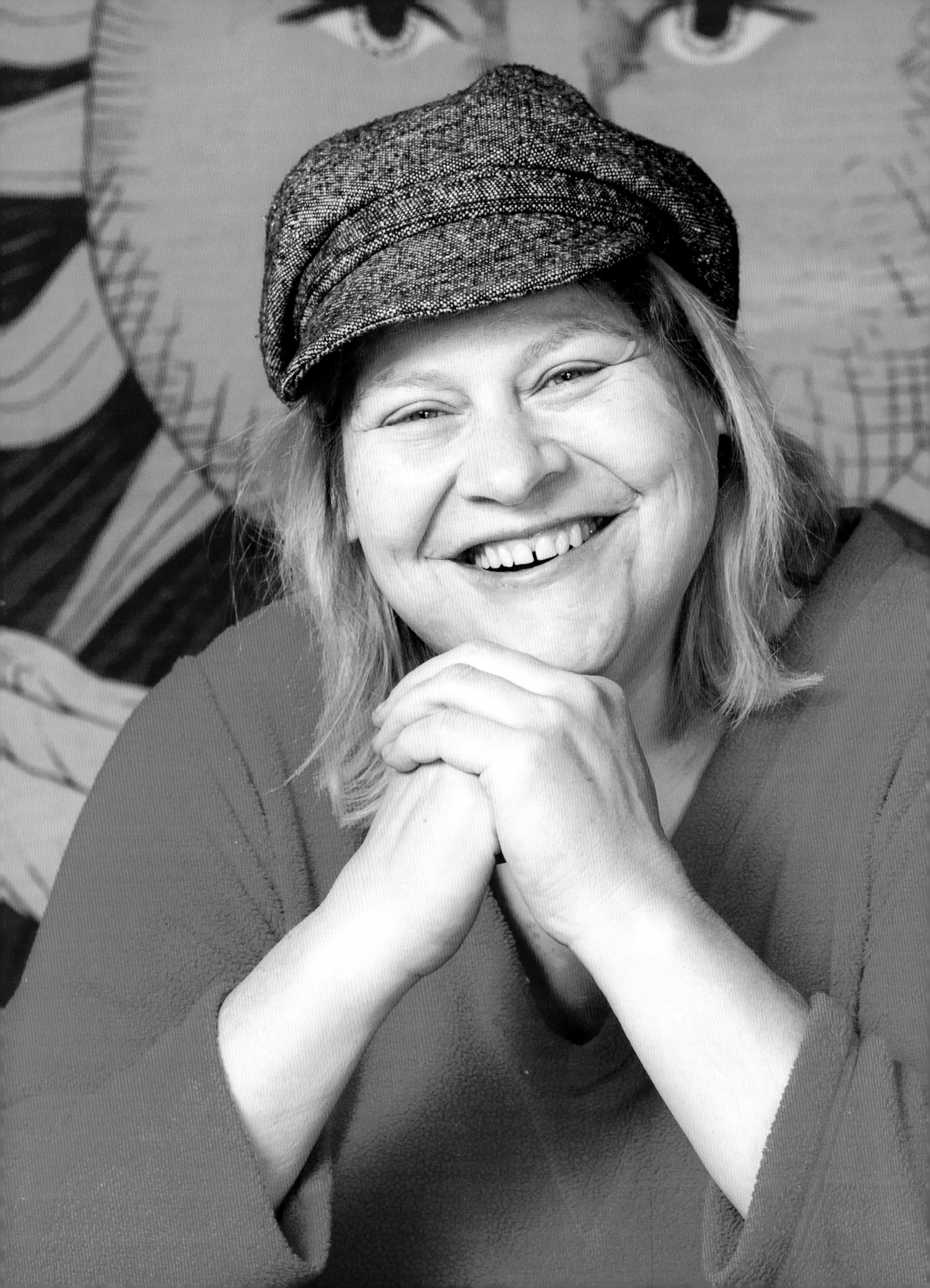

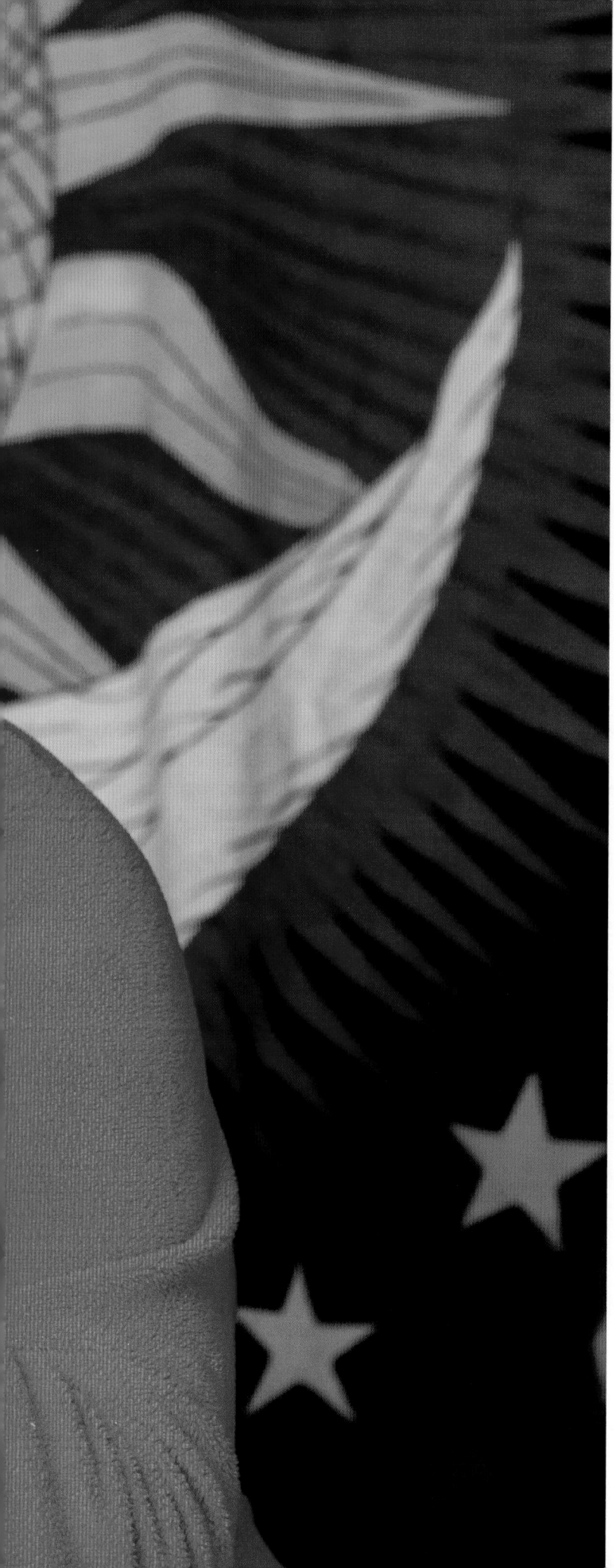

"MOSTLY, AT THIS POINT IN MY LIFE, I USE CANNABIS FOR TREATING MY PTSD. I NEED AS MUCH DISTRACTION AS POSSIBLE FOR THAT. MY BEST FRIEND WAS KILLED BY TERRORISTS."

"TAKING CBD AT NIGHT REDUCES ANXIETY BEFORE BED. EARLY AWAKENING IS A PROBLEM FOR PEOPLE WITH PTSD—YOU WAKE UP AT NIGHT AND CAN'T GET BACK TO SLEEP."

tile garden. "All of the sirens, and having to run to the shelters, sometimes 10 times a day. He deserves some childhood years of living in a peaceful, quiet place."

The blooming garden around her is bathed in early summer sun, tucked like a colorful jewel into a surrounding crown of green forest. We stepped outside to see her minuscule baby marijuana plants (all CBD cross strains of some sort), and are now en route to observe a humming bee-hive at the back of the garden. Because cannabis is state-controlled in Israel, patients can't grow it for themselves—and this contributed to Mimi's decision to move back to California, where she can exercise more control over the types she grows and uses.

"Mostly, at this point in my life, I use cannabis for treating my PTSD," she says. "I need as much distraction as possible for that. My best friend was killed by terrorists. So that's been a source of PTSD."

A beat later she adds, "I don't need to smoke very much—just a puff or two, and using a variety is critical. Changing strains almost every time I smoke is right for me."

Different types of cannabis help with different elements of PTSD, which

include avoidance, nightmares and hypersensitivity, and Mimi is experienced enough to know which to turn to at which moments. "If it's avoidance that's up for me that day, I'll sit here and think 'I cannot face the world today. I'm just going to sit in the house.' And smoking a light sativa often gives me the courage to leave, or the distraction," she explains. "For nightmares, taking CBD at night reduces anxiety before bed. Early awakening is a problem for people with PTSD—you wake up at night and can't get back to sleep. And, really, health starts with a good night's sleep, with every disease. A little bit of indica at that point will make you tired."

Mimi pauses, stooping into a chicken-wire enclosure to pluck a few blueberries from their bush. She hands one of the small indigo orbs to me and pops the other in her mouth. "Have you ever had fresh blueberries?" she asks, her tranquil new home, ripe with new beginnings, framed behind her. "I hadn't before yesterday. And now I don't think I ever really had a blueberry until I tried these."

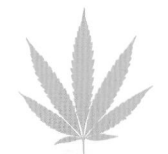

STEPHEN CLEMENTS

Age 35 / **Depression** / Nashville, Tennessee

Starting high school is a stressful milestone for any teen. For Stephen Clements, the occasion was made more dramatic by his family's move from Henry, Tennessee, a town with a population hovering around 500, to Memphis, a metropolis more than 1,000 times its size. Stephen had little in common with his new classmates, who began picking on him. Dejected and isolated, Stephen saw his peers, and the world more broadly, in a harsh, judgmental light.

"I was painfully awkward," he says. "I probably had some sort of anxiety issues looking back. Also, I came from a very hellfire-and-brimstone Southern Baptist upbringing, so while I was polite, I was an incredibly judgmental little guy. I spent a long time thinking, 'these people are bad.' I wasn't accepting of other folks."

His hostility snowballed over the years, and by the time he arrived at the University of Memphis for college, he "seethed anger all the time and had a fairly toxic inner life."

"It became apparent to me that my spirit was filled with despair," he says, "and I thought I'd never feel better than I did." In September 2001, still in his first year of college, he took a friend up on a standing offer to try marijuana—something he'd resolutely disapproved of until then.

"For the first time, I was able to take a step back from the immediacy of my problems and relax," Stephen explains. "It wasn't a miracle cure and overnight everything that was negative turned positive, but it definitely helped with the anger issues and I began my journey toward being less hostile and judgmental toward other people."

He began to see marijuana in harmony with, rather than in conflict with, his faith, and let go of his damning attitude. "I thought, 'I smoke pot and I didn't go nuts and kill anybody and I don't feel like my life is ruined now, like I have been told for years and years would happen. So if I've been lied to about that, are all these other people really as bad as they had been made out to be?' The answer was no."

The years since were embroidered with accomplishments, a trajectory Stephen attributes to his use of cannabis. He obtained bachelors and masters degrees, served in the Army (during which time he did not use cannabis), traveled the world, became a Freemason, and penned several books, including a work of historical fiction about the Byzantine Empire titled *To Save a Life*. Today, he holds a job at the Department of Veterans Affairs, is a politically active Republican eyeing a seat in local office, and lends a "clean-cut" image to the legalization movement as a member of the marijuana advocacy group Tennessee United.

All of this was possible, he says, because cannabis "got me out of the mental prison I'd built for myself, one surrounded by hostility and frustration, and got me to become part of the rest of this world."

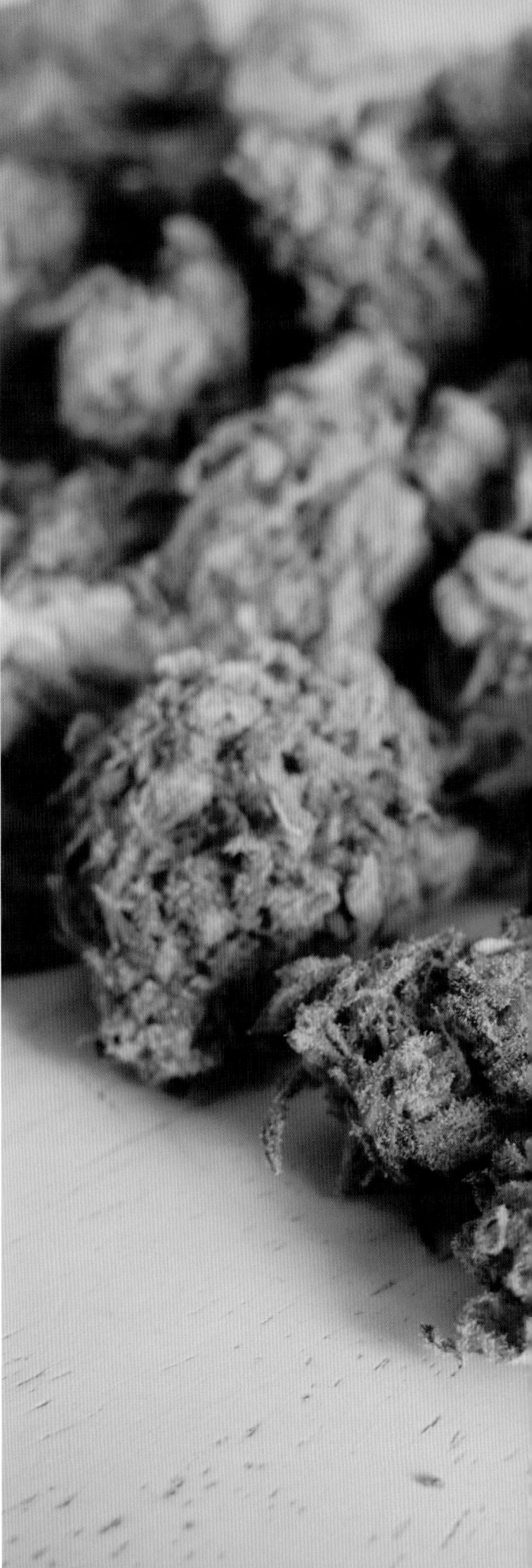

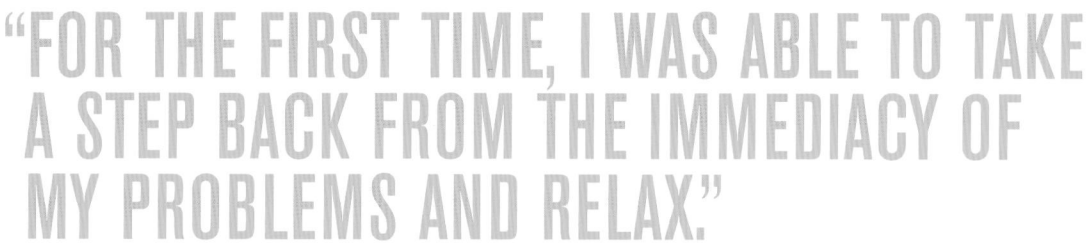

“FOR THE FIRST TIME, I WAS ABLE TO TAKE A STEP BACK FROM THE IMMEDIACY OF MY PROBLEMS AND RELAX.”

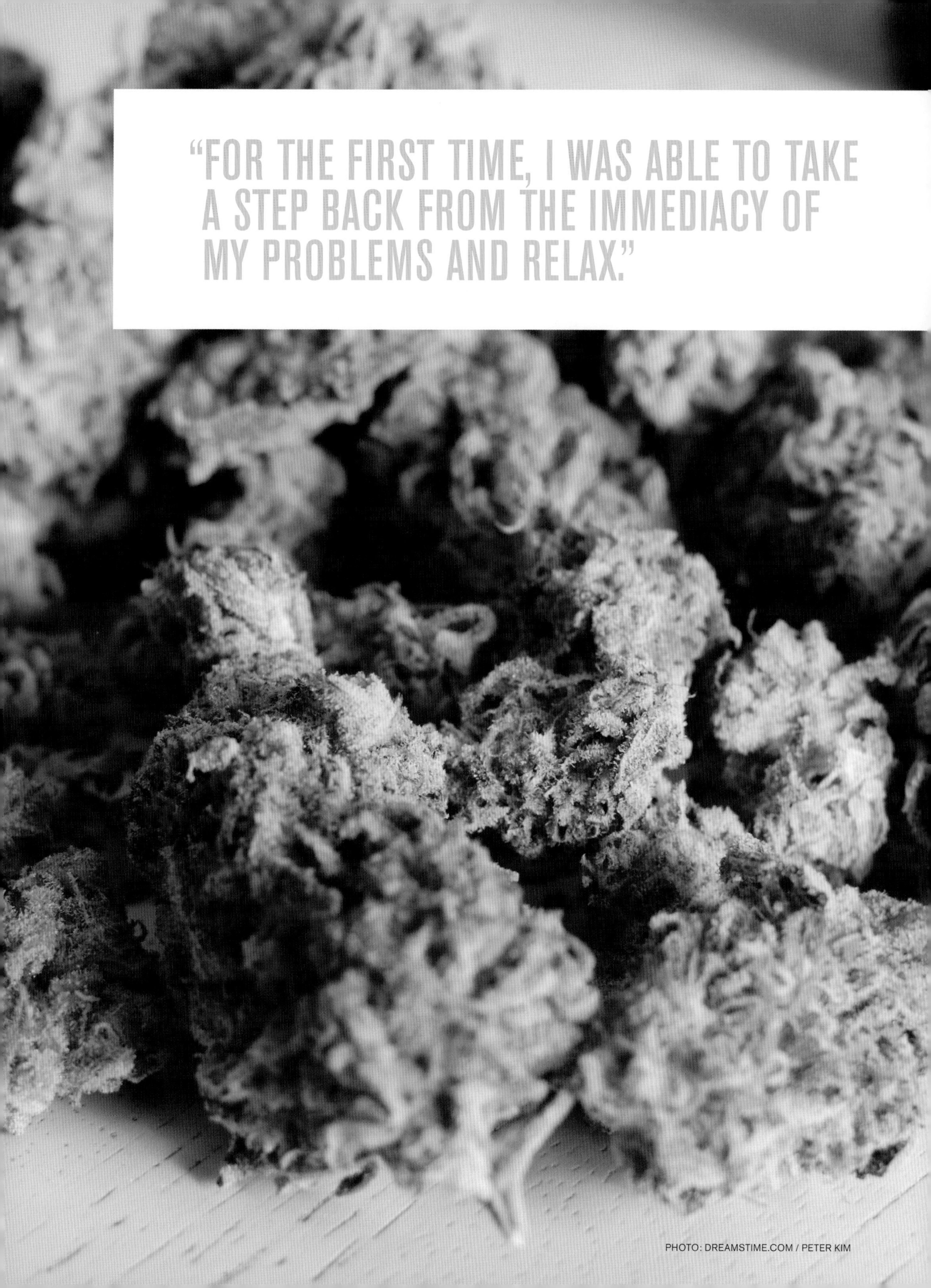

PHOTO: DREAMSTIME.COM / PETER KIM

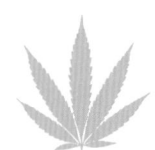

STEVEN THOMPSON

Age 67 / **Chronic Pain, Vision Problems** / Benzonia, Michigan

A s the only child of a suit-and-tie businessman growing up in Ohio, Steven Thompson joined the ranks in his family's restaurant empire, which included 10 burger joints and a dozen Kentucky Fried Chickens, by the age of 8.

In his late 20s, two decades into his involvement in the family business, Steven had a hemorrhage in his left eye. Doctors told him he had the blood pressure of an 80-year-old man and warned that he wouldn't live to see 80 if he continued with his stressful work habits. The entire family wound up retiring from the food industry in 1972, two years after which Steven moved to Manton, Michigan.

"I don't know how my dad ended up with me—I'm a country boy and I love my jeans," Steven says. "He was always in a business suit. He'd mow his lawn in dress slacks and a white shirt and tie. When I moved here in '74, and he and mom made their first trip up, he said 'you were raised to be a business professional, why are you out here where the roads aren't paved?'"

But rural life suited Steven, who moved in 1980 to the tiny village of Benzonia, Michigan, where he lives in a large turn-of-the-century farmhouse. The slower pace was kinder on his health issues, as well, which started at the age of 4 with German measles that settled in his eyes. He'd be blind by 40—that was the prognosis, although today he's 67 and still able to see well enough to drive so long as he wears his glasses. Another problem was an underactive thyroid, for which Steven, during his tenure at one of the burger restaurants, was prescribed a pill. After five sleepless days, during

"IF JESUS WERE HERE TODAY, HE'D BE TOKING RIGHT ALONG WITH US."

which he was unable to eat, he flushed the medications down the toilet and swore off prescription drugs forever.

It was out back of one of those burger eateries that an 18-year-old Steven first smoked marijuana, although he didn't understand it as medicine until he was in his 20s. He researched cannabis after moving to northern Michigan, concluding that it was "a natural herb, created by God, for our use, and it's good for you."

"To me, it's always been a plant," says Steven, who has been a Christian minister since 1984. "I don't see how you can grow a drug out of the ground. A drug to me is something man makes, not God."

He believes his cannabis use has slowed the progression of various conditions he faces, including the aforementioned vision problems and also painful arthritis in his lower back that developed in his early 40s and would leave him bedridden for a day or two at a time. Because he does not take prescription drugs, he

was told he'd have to live with that pain as it continued to worsen. But recent x-rays have shown that the arthritis has not advanced nearly as far as expected, which Steven says he owes to an increased cannabis regimen.

Cannabis's role in his own life has inspired him to advocate for the plant more widely, both as the former executive director of Michigan NORML, a nonprofit marijuana lobbying organization, and as the current chapter director of Benzie County NORML. He doesn't shy away from discussing cannabis in religious settings, either, which led to a parting of ways with the Pentecostal church through which he was a minister when he came "out of the cannabis closet" in 2000. He's now been a licensed minister through Universal Life Church for 15 years, and sees cannabis as complementary to the Bible's messages. "If Jesus were here today, he'd be toking right along with us," he says.

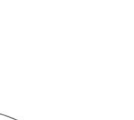

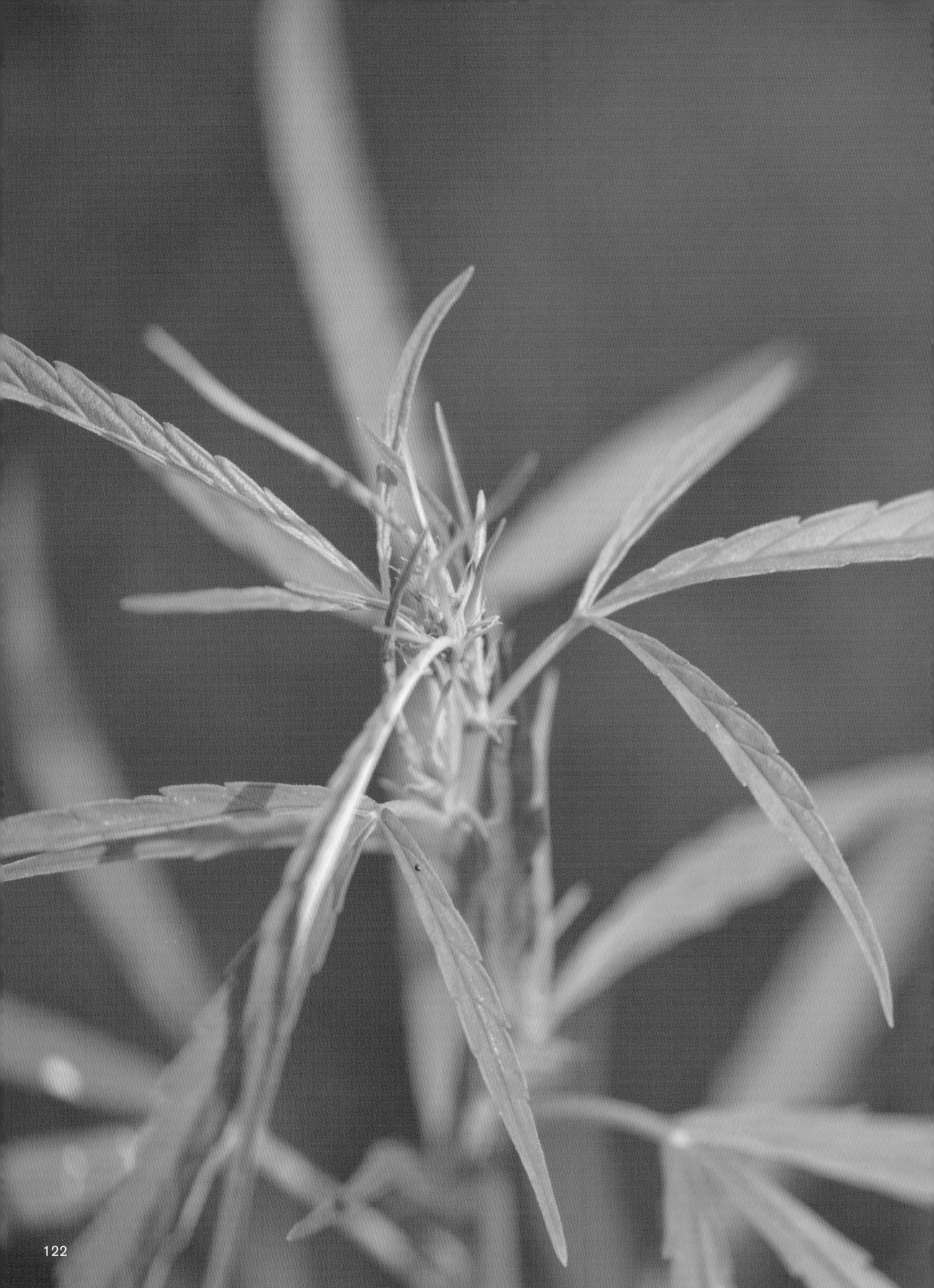

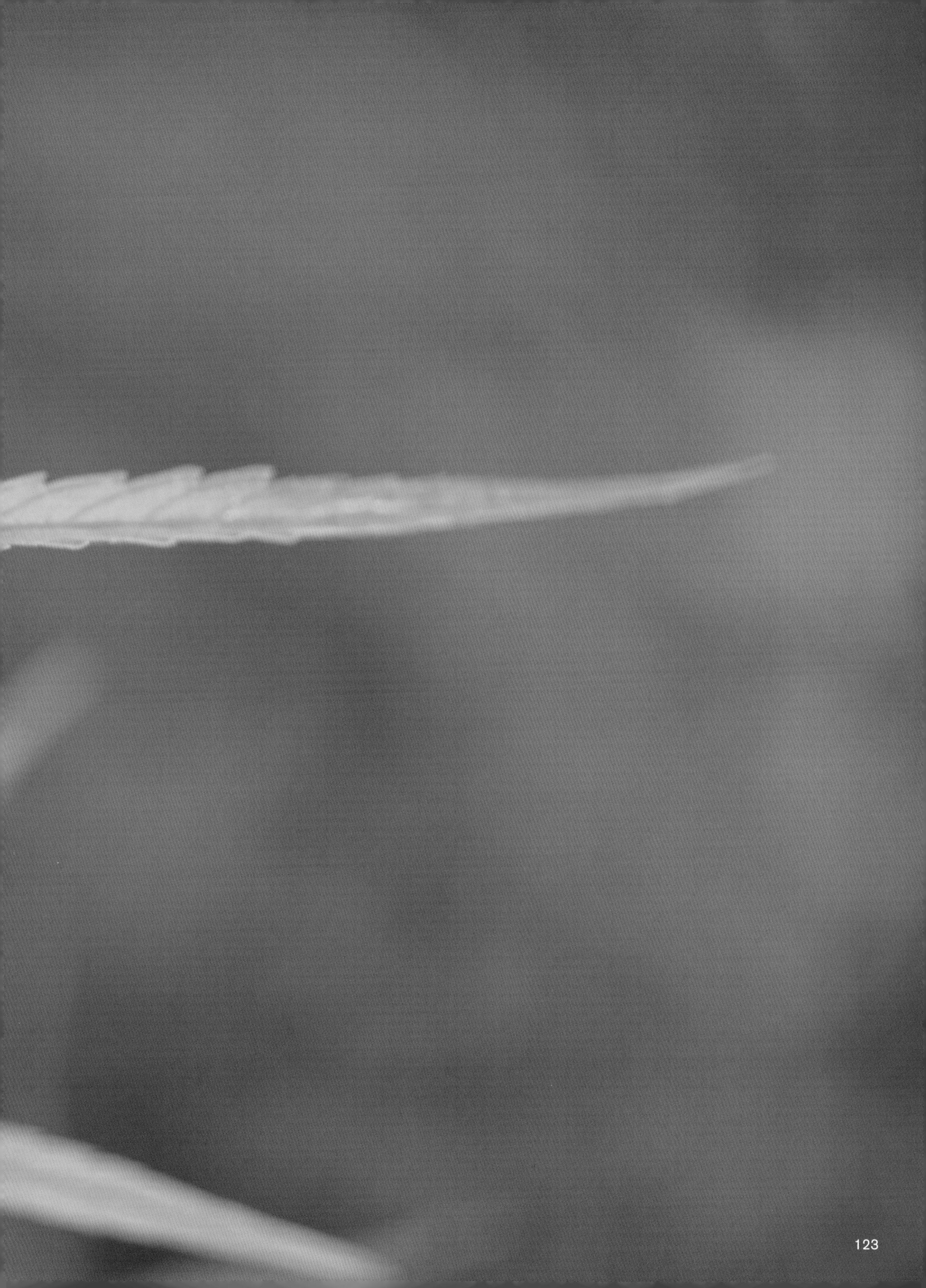

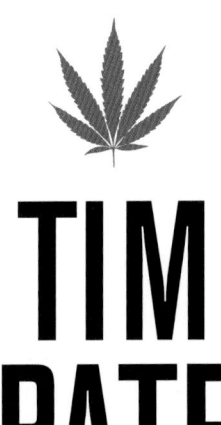

TIM PATE

Age 60 / Degenerative Bone Disease, Severe Obstructive Lung Disease, Chronic Pain / Portland, Oregon

When it's all tallied up, Tim Pate spent more than a year of his life in the hospital by the time he was 20.

His myriad health problems started early, with a severe asthma attack at the age of 5 that resulted in a two-week hospitalization. Asthma-related issues persisted for the Tulsa-raised boy, who also tested positive to allergies for 87 different things. He sustained a string of injuries and five concussions over the years, adding to his health woes. There was, for example, the bike accident in fourth grade, when he hit a fire hydrant and got a concussion, and the time in 1989 when his pickup truck rolled and he broke a shoulder.

The seemingly innocuous injury that would prove most burdensome in the long run occurred in 1986, when Tim twisted his ankle playing volleyball. "One thing led to another over the years," he says. "One tumor developed and then a couple more developed, every one of them in a bad spot."

Between 1990 and 1997, Tim was almost always having, preparing for, or recovering from surgery on his tumorous ankle, culminating with a total fusion in 1997, in which "hardware" like pins and screws were surgically implemented. One week before relaying his story, Tim had x-rays taken of the ankle that showed great improvement. But if it's not the ankle, it's always something else. At the time of this interview, Tim had undergone two abdominal surgeries in

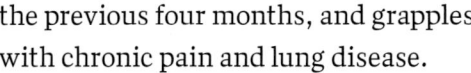
the previous four months, and grapples with chronic pain and lung disease.

He uses marijuana—by eating it, smoking it, vaporizing it, or via topical products—to manage his many ailments. "My day is livable because of cannabis," he states.

In the years leading up to his foray into using medicinal cannabis, Tim built a robust résumé in the field of crisis support. A minister with the Church of Christ at the time, he directed a crisis center for pregnant teenagers, worked in the drug-free youth movement and in drug crisis care, and served as a chairman of the board for a medical center that had a clinic for the homeless and a suicide crisis program. In 1988, he was asked to run the "down tent"—the medical station that dealt with overdoses—at Grateful Dead shows, which he did as a volunteer until Jerry Garcia's death in 1995.

"I've seen the effects of drugs on people," he says. "In all those years I never saw an OD on marijuana. Ever. And having been on the frontlines, and having been exposed to so many people, I was still straight. I wasn't sneaking off and smoking."

That changed when his father had a heart attack in 1989. Tim went home to Oklahoma, where his younger sister urged him to unwind and handed him a joint.

"I hadn't smoked since college," Tim remembers. "Suddenly, I could breathe. All the tension in my shoulders was gone. Physically, things just got better for me

because of one hit on a joint." The occasion inspired Tim to look into cannabis from a medical standpoint. Because of his numerous allergies, he wasn't able to use many pain medications, and cannabis had potential to fill that gap. "I am allergic to morphine, and too much Advil makes me bleed. Aleve puts me to sleep. There are so many pain meds out there that I can't take. I'm in a lot of pain every day, especially in the ankle and my neck, so what am I supposed to do?"

As he continued to use cannabis once he returned home to Oregon, where he has lived since 1986, he found that it not only reduced pain levels and relaxed his muscles, but also acted as an expectorant and opened up his lungs.

"It was an immediate feeling of 'Oh my God, I can breathe,'" he says. "Breathing is a big deal for an asthmatic. An asthmatic fights for every breath."

Driven by years of experience in health crisis work, in which he saw first-hand that marijuana wasn't the dangerous drug the "Just Say No" crusade made it out to be, and his newfound personal understanding of its medicinal benefits, Tim started speaking out about medical cannabis and became involved in the movement to legalize it.

"I knew what was going on," he says. "I knew how many PCP attacks there were, and the trouble with cocaine and crack at the time. And how many heroin deaths [our area] had. Those were stats we kept when I was in the business. I had

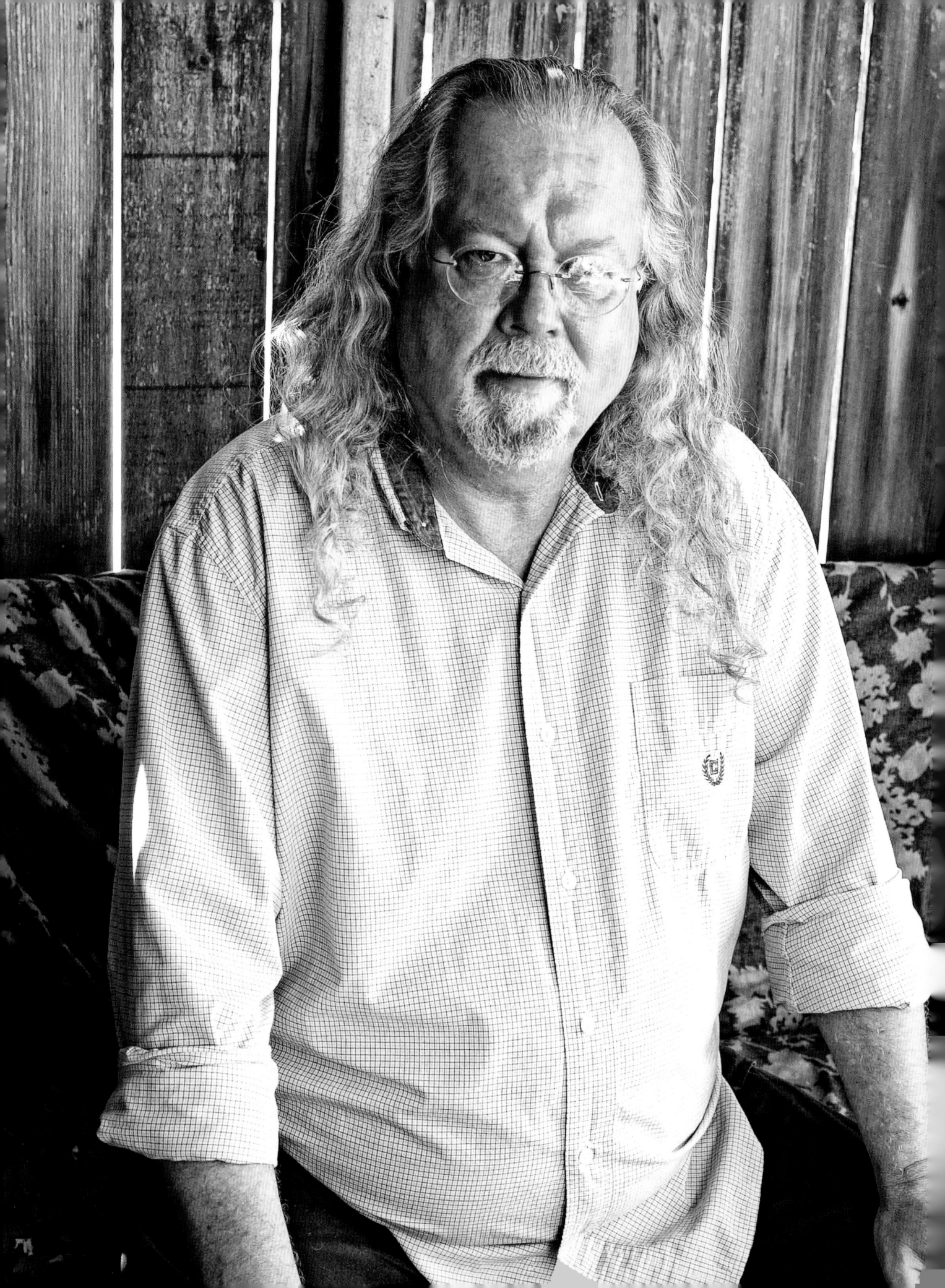

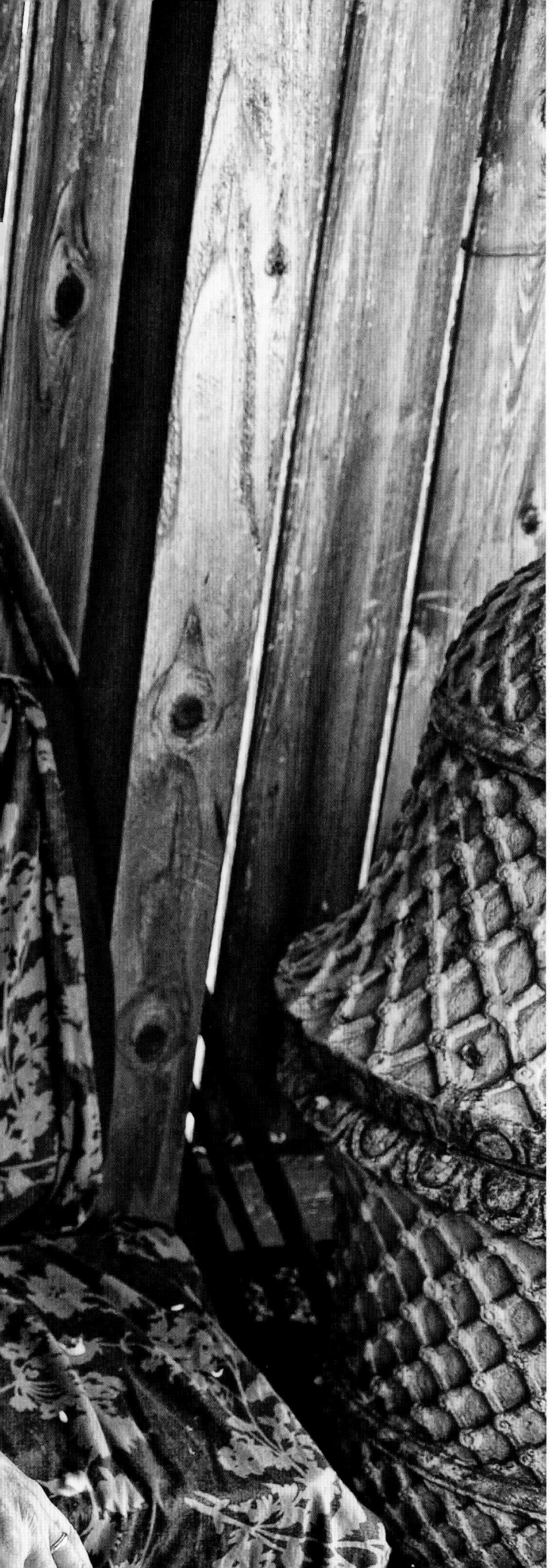

"MY DAY IS LIVABLE BECAUSE OF CANNABIS."

insider insight into what is and isn't a problem. And marijuana wasn't a problem. When I see something being treated like a problem when it isn't, I must act. I became very active."

Tim was part of Oregon's first medical marijuana efforts in the early '90s, helping to change public opinion and public policy, in that order, in the years since. Today, medical marijuana dispensaries pepper the state, and new frontiers in the cannabis and hemp industries are on the horizon, the latter of which Tim champions as a member of a state committee formed to administer hemp production.

On top of his vocal advocacy, he has spun a prolific career as a glass blower, sculptor, musician, and world-champion pumpkin carver (visit timpate. com to see his work), and cannabis, he says, has made it all possible.

PHOTO BY DARRYL YU

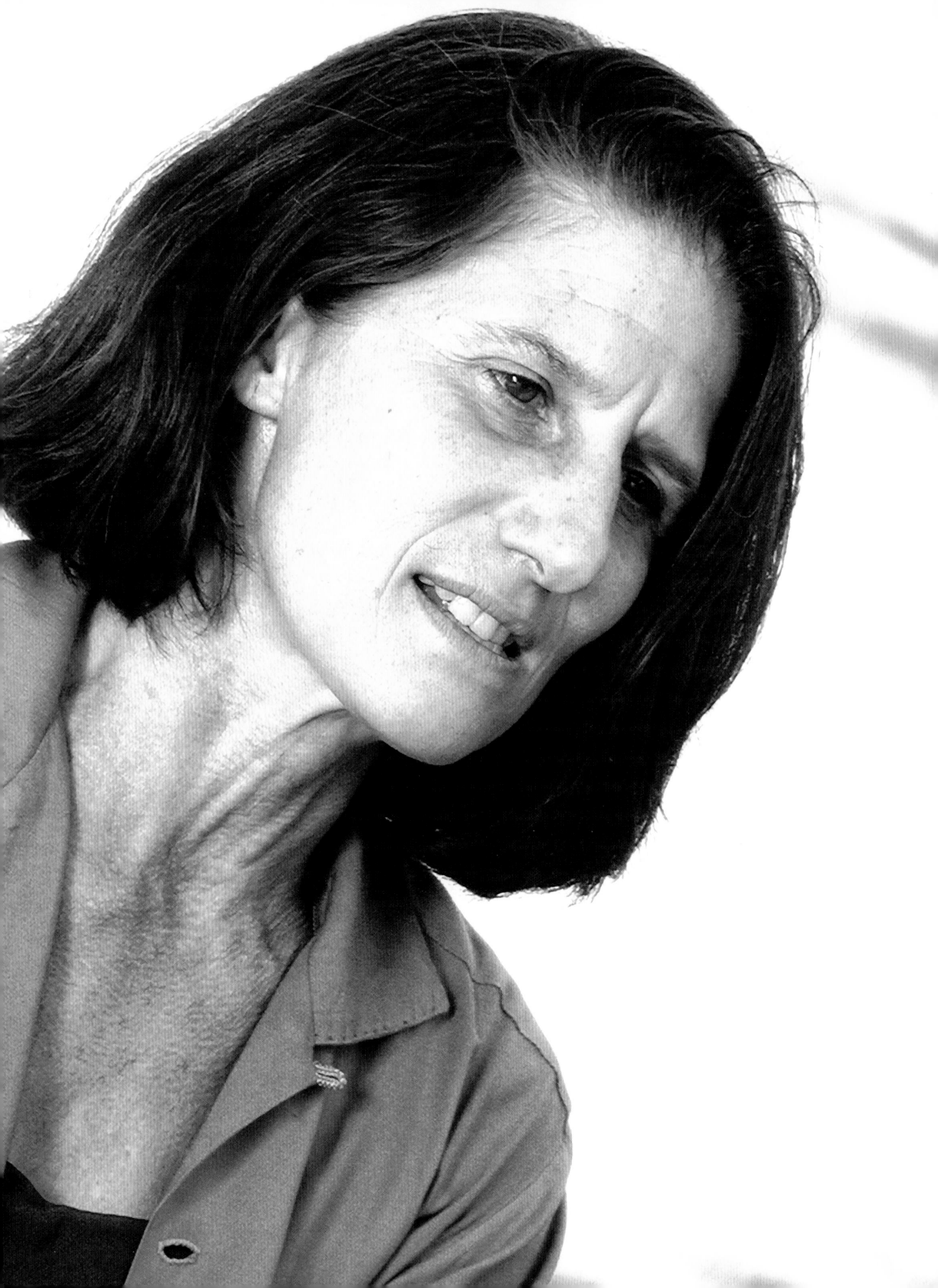

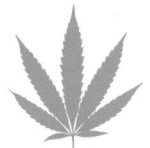

VALERIE LEVERONI CORRAL

Age 63 / **Epilepsy** / Santa Cruz County, California

The headquarters for the Wo/Men's Alliance for Medical Marijuana (WAMM) is tucked off of an industrial block in Santa Cruz, California's Westside neighborhood, 10 miles from the collective's medical marijuana farm.

The office is traced on one side by train tracks that head northwest out of town, snaking toward expanses of farm fields. In the other direction, across a sprawl of houses, locals surf world-famous waves at Steamer Lane. An "Open" sign hangs in the center of the red-framed front door, welcoming WAMM members and, on one brisk spring day, this inquiring writer.

Inside, the office is abuzz with activity, and at the center of the hive is the queen bee: Valerie Leveroni Corral, the spirited leader who founded WAMM along with her then-husband Mike Corral in 1993. Members and staff flit down the hallway and lean through doorways, showering her with questions and reminders. Two women are stationed at computers in the entryway, adding a pitter-patter of keystrokes to the soundtrack.

"Busy day," I remark as I take a seat in the waiting area.

"Oh, this is mild," says one of the women, sporting a shiny purple blouse and long gray ponytail. "You'd think dealing with medical marijuana that this would be a mellow place, but we have nearly 1,000 members and there's a lot to do."

These members are sick or dying, so there's no time to waste, she adds, and the rapidity of Valerie's responses, perceptible as they drift into the lobby, attests to that. But the routine hubbub has an undercurrent of fresh distress: as the local newspapers reported that morning, the country's longest-running medical marijuana collective was in danger of closing. With the finalization of Valerie's and Mike's divorce, the non-profit needs to raise enough money to buy the private land on which its cannabis is grown. As of this writing, WAMM was nearly $30,000 into its initial $150,000 fundraising campaign on the crowd-sourcing website Indiegogo.

"We're trying to raise more than a million dollars all together," Valerie tells me in her office a few minutes later. As I sink onto a teal couch, amidst leopard print pillows and a throw blanket, she finishes shuffling through a stack of paperwork, slipping them into open filing cabinet drawers. She's standing beside her desk, where an exercise ball is parked in lieu of a chair. When she joins me on the couch, her petite frame is accentuated by the stretch of hardwood floors, white walls, and the crowded bookcase

behind her. A title stands out among the rest: *How We Die.*

THE CRASH

In 1973, Valerie was an energetic 20-year-old living in Squaw Valley, California, on the northwestern shore of Lake Tahoe. She had dreams of becoming a doctor, and was working in a research lab while studying art and philosophy at the University of Nevada in Reno.

One day, she sat in the passenger seat of her gray Volkswagen Bug as a girlfriend steered it down the open desert highway that leads to Pyramid Lake, an oasis in an otherwise barren desert where, years later, the experimental art festival Burning Man found a home. A restored P51 fighter plane appeared, heading toward the car at such a low height that Valerie's friend could see the pilot's moustache.

"We thought he must need to land, so we decided to pull off and wait,'" she says, ignoring the ringing phone on her desk. The World War II aircraft

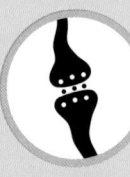 **ENDOCANNABINOID SYSTEM:** The human body is built to respond to cannabis through what is called the endocannabinoid system, comprised of cannabinoid receptors in the brain and throughout the body. Humans and other animals naturally produce substances to stimulate the cannabinoid receptors, which are essential to maintaining the body's internal systems and helping us respond to ever changing and sometimes dangerous outside stimuli. The endocannabinoid system regulates numerous functions, such as inflammatory responses and the recycling of cell materials, and is important for controlling pain, promoting healing and marshaling anti-tumor responses. Numerous compounds in marijuana, such as THC and CBD, also stimulate our cannabinoid receptors, which is thought to be why cannabis has so many medicinal applications. Scientists are still working to broaden our understanding of how the endocannabinoid system works, but it's become clear that it is essential to maintaining good health. *Source: NORML.*

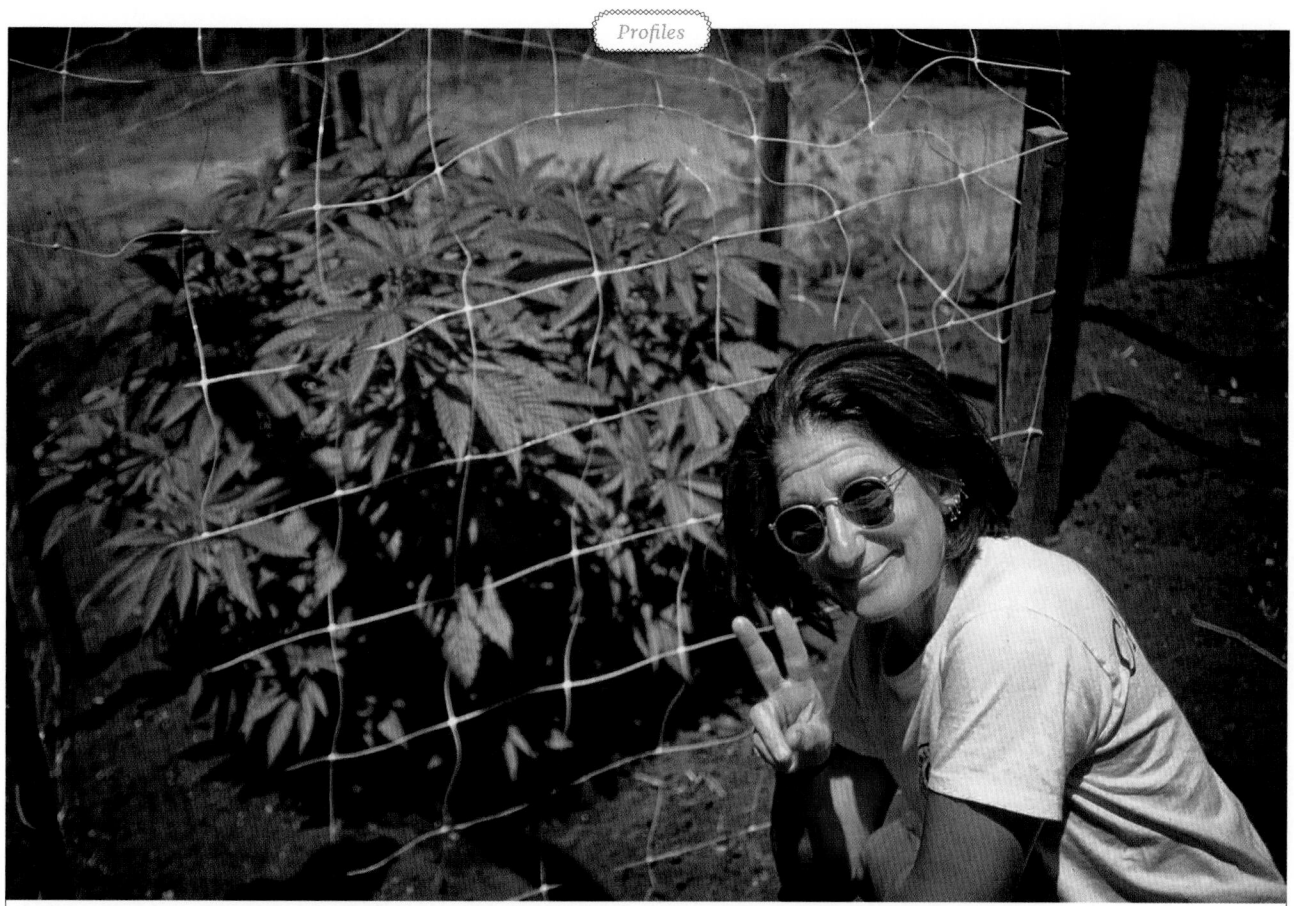

THE PLANE ZOOMED OVER THE BUG FROM BEHIND SO FAST AND SO LOW THAT THE FORCE TOSSED THE CAR INTO THE AIR.

whooshed overhead, circled the lake, and zoomed back over the Bug from behind so fast and so low that the force tossed the car into the air. It crashed down and rolled for the length of a football field, coming to a halt with Valerie splayed partially outside of the car, unconscious from a head injury, and her friend thrown off to the side.

In a fateful display of luck, an off-duty deputy witnessed the accident from where he and his son were collecting arrowheads in the desert. He called it in on his two-way radio, but it was 45 minutes before help arrived on scene. Valerie was taken to a hospital in Reno and released the next day—but something wasn't right.

"I was pretty out of it," says Valerie, who lived alone at the time. "I'd wake up with my tongue bitten, or having fallen, but not understanding what was happening."

Valerie leans forward as she speaks, bending one of her jean- and boot-clad legs and bringing it onto the couch. Her dark, red-tinted hair is pulled back into a ponytail, revealing a row of gold hoop earrings that adorn her left ear.

She recalls how, after the accident, she had to study much harder than usual and was struggling to function normally. It wasn't until a friend saw her have a seizure that she had a word for what was happening to her. She was hospitalized again, this time for several weeks, and diagnosed with grand mal seizures as a result of her traumatic brain injury. Doctors sent her home with a menu of prescriptions to help her manage—strong anticonvulsants, Valium, and Percodan, among them.

Between five grand mal seizures a day and the prescription-induced fog, her life lost all semblance of what it was like before.

"I couldn't function anymore," she says. "It was like living under water. I couldn't leave the house. When you have an illness, your life is different. And often the illness is at the core of your daily life. Everything that was normal is different. You have a new normal. Now your life is about making it to the bathroom or not having a grand mal seizure."

She left college and moved to California, where she and Mike settled into a rustic home in the Santa Cruz Mountains. Surrounded by a redwood forest, Valerie felt more at ease than in the city, and bolstered her quality of life by enjoying nature, growing her own food, and eating a vegetarian diet.

Decades before Google brought medical research to our fingertips, the couple learned about her condition in medical journals, where, in 1974, Mike stumbled across an abstract that discussed cannabis as a treatment for epilepsy in mice. Intrigued and desperate for an effective medicine, Valerie gave it a try, keeping a log of the usage.

"Within three-and-a-half weeks, I noticed neurological differences," she says. "Not gone, but markedly reduced, so much so that I could trust change was happening."

Soon the duo was growing and breeding the plant, experimenting with strains to find the best possible treatment for Valerie's epilepsy. "It took a long time to get off the pharmaceuticals because I was addicted to them," she notes.

The seizures went away entirely after two-and-a-half years, although she still has "some neurological issues." She doesn't hesitate to say that cannabis was what healed her: "It saved my life," she states.

THE ROAD TO WAMM

After several brushes with law enforcement for growing marijuana, the Corrals decided to band together with other patients to form a collective. Since 1993, WAMM has grown and produced marijuana (indicas, sativas, and hybrids), tinctures, edibles, salves, and capsules—all lab tested for quality and potency—that is free to its members in exchange for participation, as they are able, in WAMM operations.

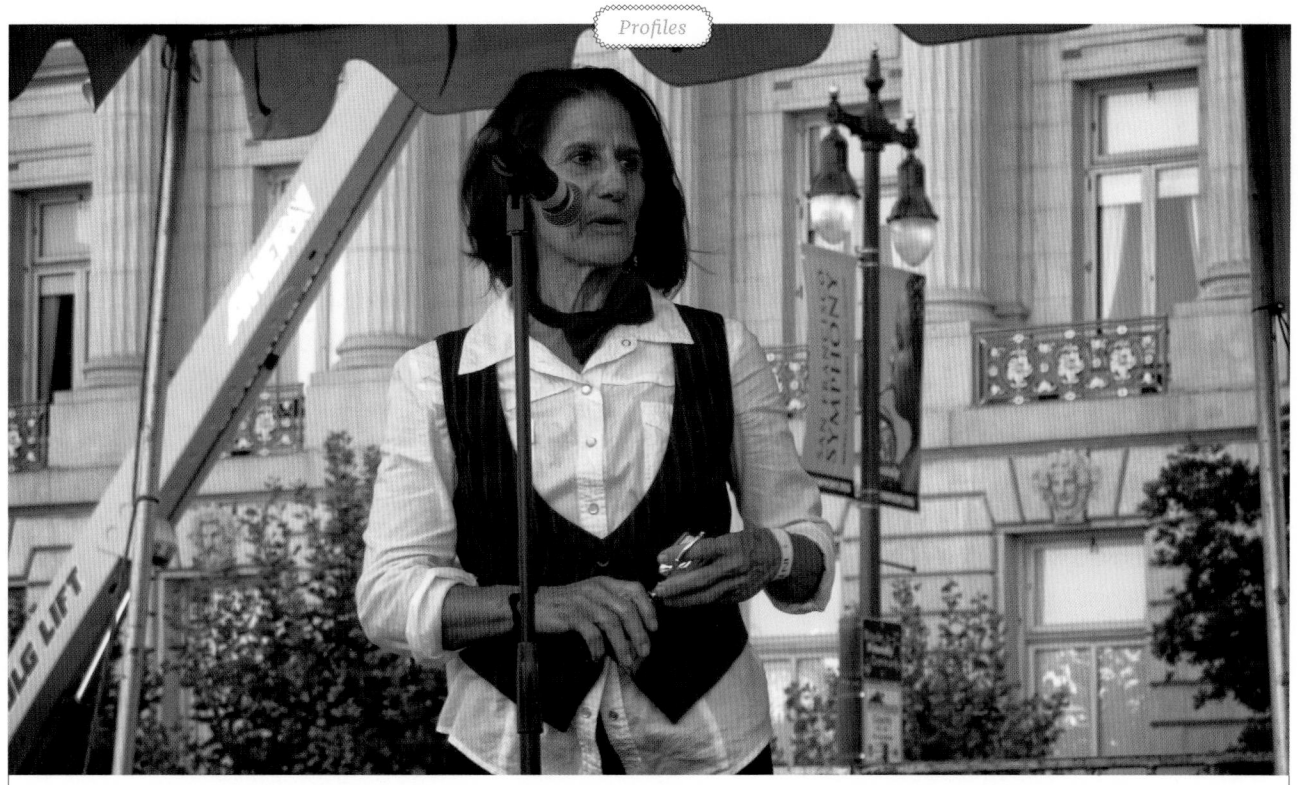

"WHEN YOU HAVE AN ILLNESS, YOUR LIFE IS DIFFERENT. AND OFTEN THE ILLNESS IS AT THE CORE OF YOUR DAILY LIFE. EVERYTHING THAT WAS NORMAL IS DIFFERENT. YOU HAVE A NEW NORMAL."

"Building WAMM came out of a Marxist principle—it's a basic tribal principle, really: from each according to his ability, to each according to his need," Valerie explains, unclasping her hands to gesture for emphasis. "You do what you can, give what you can, take what you need."

The DEA infamously raided the WAMM garden in 2002, after which the organization successfully sued the federal government and was deputized by local law enforcement to ensure they could continue providing medicine to sick and dying residents in peace.

Cancer is the most common illness among WAMM'S members, who number more than 800 (150 to 200 of whom are participating at any given time), although Valerie lists ALS, Parkinson's, multiple sclerosis, and more as other life-threatening conditions they often see.

Whatever a person's condition, Valerie draws on her own experience with illness in her relationships with WAMM members. "You don't have to suffer to do good things, but when you have, it changes the way you engage with another person who is suffering," she says.

She understands how an illness minimizes one's life. How it changes the day-to-day things and the big-picture things, too. Crucially, she remembers what it was like for family and friends to be uncomfortable around her.

Being there for a sick person is about "knowing how to be still and allowing someone else to have their experience without feeling like you have to change it," she says. "It's about being OK with your discomfort when witnessing someone else's suffering. To learn from it."

A BEARER OF PEACE

When Valerie's own father was dying, in 1989, a friend told her, "Healing is not always of the body, but it's always of the spirit."

She appreciates this now in ways she didn't yet then. Today, she's been at the bedside of more than 150 WAMM members as they have left this world and says "it's shifted the way I feel about healing."

For WAMM's terminal patients, for whom physical healing isn't the point, cannabis brings relief of a different sort: the alleviation of pain, suffering and anxiety in the face of death.

The first time of many that Valerie witnessed cannabis usher in a tranquil death was in 1998. "It was the first time I was present with a person where I became aware that cannabis was really an effec-

tive tool when someone was dying, as they were *actually* dying," she says.

"One of our members had gone into that coma-like state that can precede death," she goes on. "There was a nurse there. The family was very uptight, and there was a schism and problems between the patient and them, and to them cannabis was … "—here, she cringes dramatically to evoke their disdain for the plant.

"I rolled a joint and did what is called a shotgun, where you turn the joint around and you blow in on his in-breath."

After three breaths, the man smiled a tiny smile and gave a thumbs up.

"He passed away, but he came to for about five to seven hours," Valerie recalls. "He was conscious, and the family healed a lot in their conversation."

More than 20 years later, she's lost count of the number of patients who have said cannabis—particularly the oils—has eased their dread about dying.

"It's opened a door to accepting death and quelled their fear about the process," Valerie says. "It allows people to engage, to expand their consciousness—which is a very important thing if you're dying, because that's probably what you're going to need to use to quell fear of the unknown. When they have been able to engage in that experience, their deaths have been profoundly peaceful."

THE COMPLEXITY OF HEALING

Valerie's insights into cannabis's capacity for physical healing are just as

"HEALING IS SO COMPLEX. IT'S NOT JUST ONE THING. YOU DON'T HEAL BECAUSE SOMEONE SHOOTS YOU UP WITH A PHARMACEUTICAL, OTHERWISE EVERYONE WOULD BE BETTER, WOULDN'T THEY?"

rich, culled from more than two decades at the helm of WAMM, as well as her personal experience. Her main takeaway: "That every human is a unique universe, totally different from the next person."

"The reason cannabis—like many other plants—works is because we evolved with it," she explains. "And that evolution is part of the symbiotic relationship of healing for living in and on and of the planet."

She cites one of "hundreds and hundreds" of examples, a story about two WAMM members who both had Stage 4 Non-Small Cell Lung Cancer. One used a high-CBD, low-THC medication. "The other comes in—same disease, same prognosis—and does high THC and very little CBD," Valerie says. "After three to five months, both have no evidence of disease."

Cannabis, when approached the WAMM way, is effective because it is adaptable to a person's needs. Different strains, methods, ratios, dosages—these are all considered as WAMM works with each member to develop an individualized protocol. The organization treats

cannabis as one piece in a toolkit that includes environment, attitude, diet, and alternative or conventional treatments and medicines of a person's choice.

Because of this intricacy, Valerie is worried about what will happen when—and she says it is a matter of *when*, not *if*—cannabis is coopted by Big Pharma.

"The pharmaceutical industry, being a business rather than [being] focused on healing, doesn't have room for us—it doesn't have room for nature, because you can't patent nature," she says. "They need to tweak it to own it, to make it into something they can sell."

The result, she believes, will be that a multifaceted plant will be homogenized and reduced into limited dosages. "So it won't have the extremely potent effectiveness and outcome that we're finding now," Valerie laments. The pursuit of profit will take the plant further and further from its full capacity.

"Healing is so complex," she says. "It's not just one thing. You don't heal because someone shoots you up with a pharmaceutical, otherwise everyone would be better, wouldn't they?"

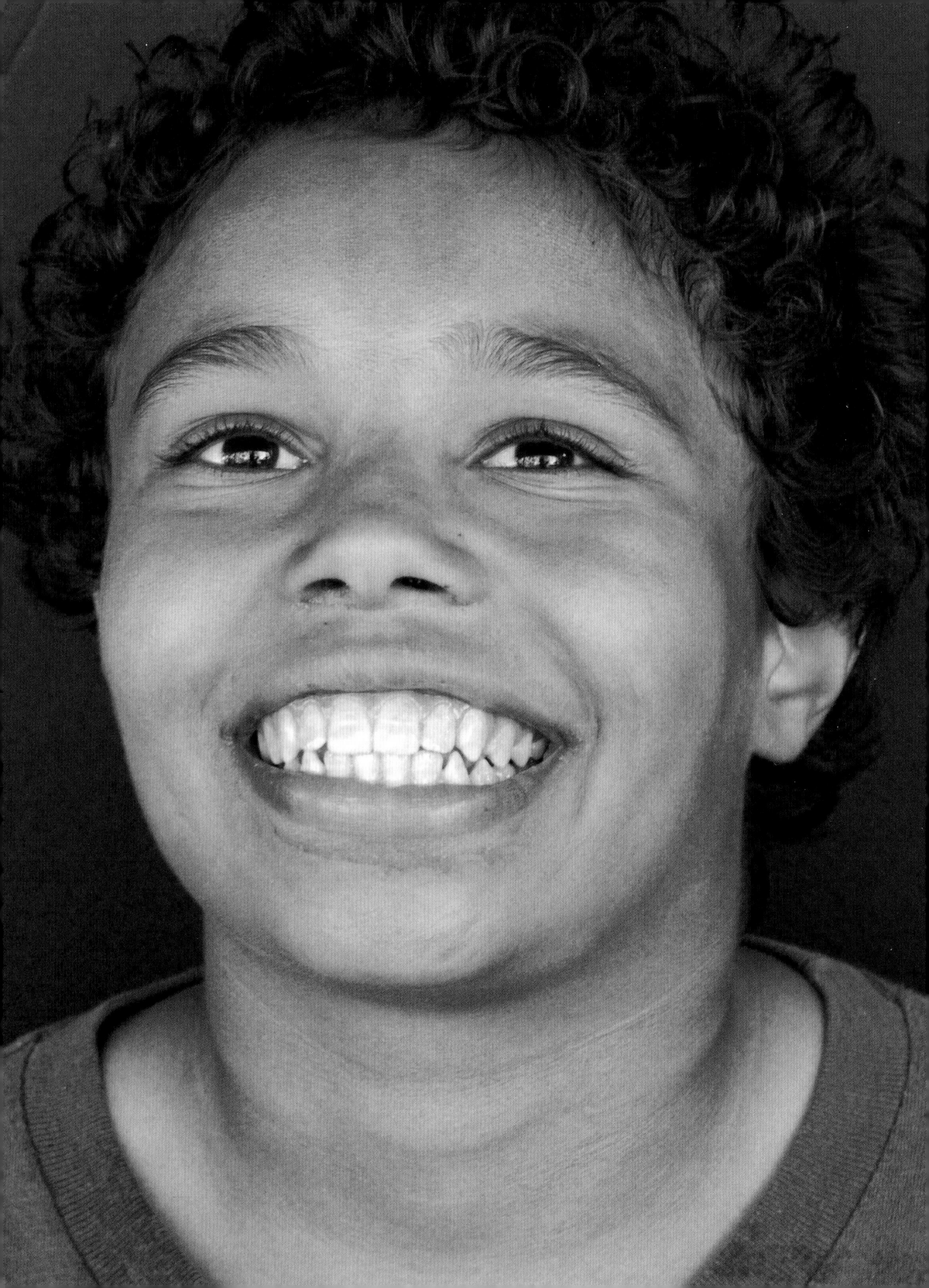

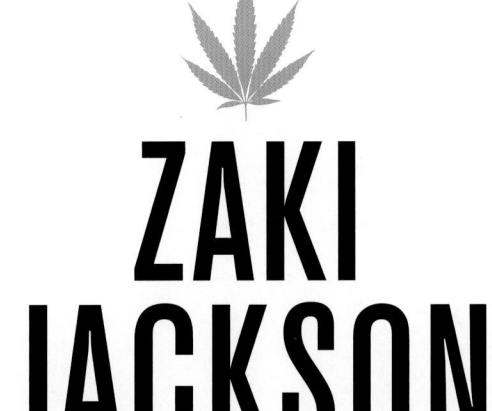

ZAKI JACKSON

Age 12 / **Doose Syndrome** / Colorado Springs, Colorado

The first thing Heather Jackson did each day for much of her son Zaki's life was make sure he was still alive.

It all started in September of 2003, when Zaki was just 4 months old. The infant began having strange episodes that baffled his parents. His small body would clench up, and he'd throw his head back. If he was holding a rattle, it was often flicked up into the air. Sometimes it occurred in response to loud noises, leading Heather to believe her son was easily startled.

But it was happening quite a bit by the time Zaki was 6 months old, when doctors took his first electroencephalogram (EEG), a diagnostic test for epilepsy.

"When the doctor's office called, it was the doctor, not the nurse or the receptionist," recalls Heather. "So I figured it was bad. He said it was seizures."

Around 15 months old, Zaki (pronounced zah-kai) was diagnosed with Doose Syndrome, or Myoclonic-Astatic Epilepsy (MAE), a rare, little-understood and grave form of early child-onset epilepsy that is often irresponsive to medication.

The condition progressed to the point, in 2011, where Zaki was having hundreds of brief, violent seizures a day. As his mom puts it, "his brain was under constant assault for the better part of a decade."

For years, he had also experienced what are called non-convulsive status episodes, which aren't necessarily visible seizures, at least not as most people would recognize them.

"But the brain is in seizure activity," explains Heather. "He'd dip into this status where he'd stop talking and walking; he would lose his swallow reflex. These could last a day, a couple of days, a couple of weeks." If the halt on talking, walking and swallowing continued, Heather and her husband, Frank, had to feed him fluids through a syringe.

They never knew when the spell would break and who he would be when it did. Years of seizures translated into significant delays—the "collateral damage," in Heather's words—that put Zaki at 28 to 41 months old developmentally. A persistent parade of weekly occupational, speech and physical therapies helped some, but any progress could be washed away by a single episode.

"It would set him back months developmentally and all of the hard work we did every day was just gone," Heather says. "I'd crumble, give up, scream, yell and kick, and then I'd get up in the morning and brush myself off and say, because of him, we've gotta continue on."

CHERISHING THEIR TIME

In the fall of 2011, Zaki began having chronic seizures called tonics in which he'd cease breathing. Every time it happened, a part of Heather feared it was the end. She awoke every day and habitually looked over to him, where he slept in his parents' bed or nearby on a makeshift bed on the floor. (Attempts at normalcy—by having him in his own room, albeit

with a pulse oximeter monitoring machine—never stuck.) As 2011 came to a close, it seemed that Zaki's young life would, as well. The family took a Make-A-Wish trip to Disneyworld and tried to cherish the time they had left together.

"We were doing the best we could," says Heather. "We were enjoying him. We were not focused on death. We were focused on living and trying to be happy. But it's hard when the first thing you do in the morning is check your kid to see if he still has a pulse. It's a really difficult way to live."

After 17 pharmaceuticals were tried, and failed, Zaki's doctors didn't have anything left in their bag of tricks.

"Our option was to recycle through the drugs we'd tried, which was definitely not something I was interested in doing," says Heather. "Every pharmaceutical has side effects, and the drugs they use to control epilepsy are really heavy hitting."

Some drugs diminished Zaki's appetite; others made him eat too much. Some caused him to lose sleep; others forced him to sleep all day. He didn't sweat the entire two-and-a-half year period he was taking Topamax.

"The most successful, long-term therapy he tried was steroids," his mother adds. "Zaki has bone loss, cataracts. He's like an old man because of these pharmaceuticals."

TURNING TO CANNABIS

Zaki's initial diagnosis, nearly a decade earlier, had kicked off an "affair with research" for Heather. Fueled by the fury and fervor of a desperate parent, she investigated every possible treatment and proposed medication. And as each failed to bring her little boy out of the dark, one unexplored option flickered promisingly in the distance.

Swinging her researcher's spotlight onto cannabis, though, meant overcoming her personal hang-ups.

"This is your brain on drugs." Like many others who grew up in the 1980s, that was the no-nonsense message—

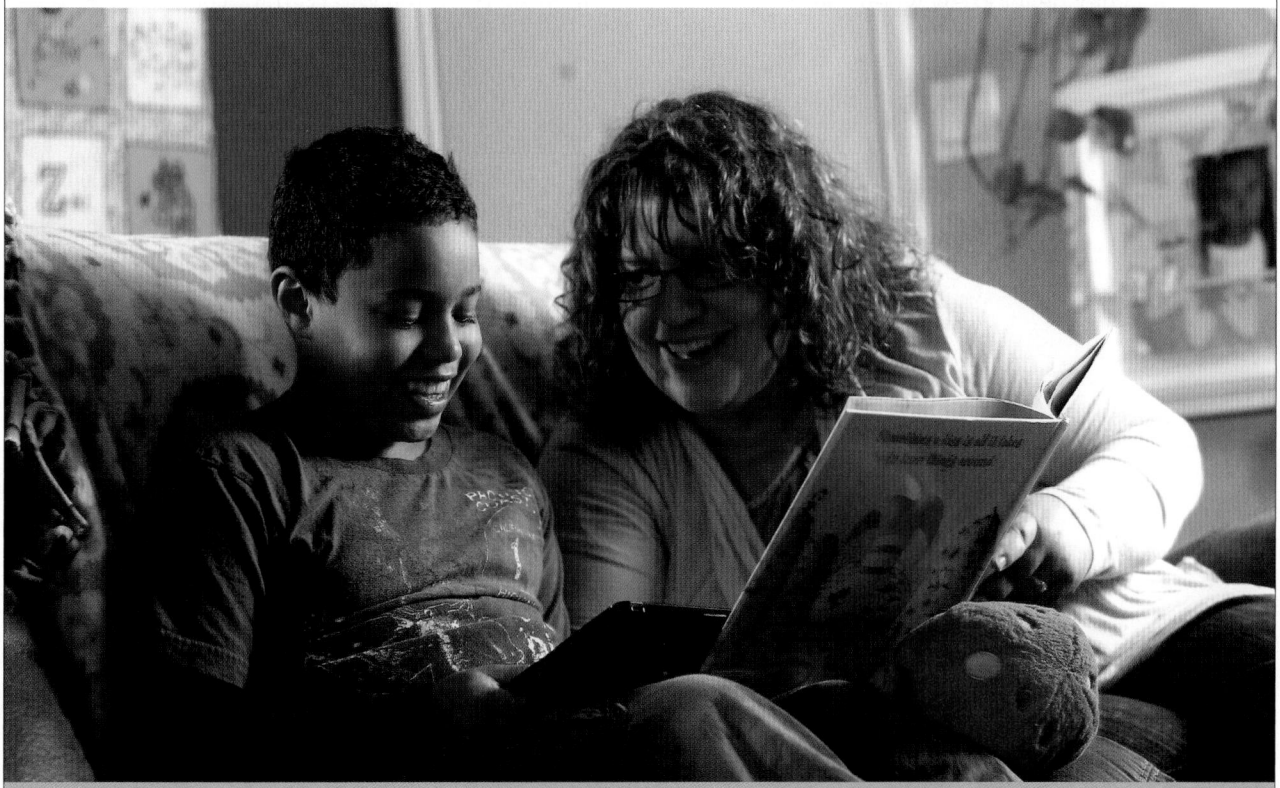

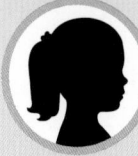 **CHARLOTTE'S WEB:** Charlotte's Web is a form of non-psychoactive cannabis oil used to treat seizures in children. The oil was named after Charlotte Figi, a 5-year-old girl who suffered from uncontrollable epileptic seizures. The only treatment that worked was a certain strain of CBD oil, which her mother said stopped 99.9 percent of the seizures. After Charlotte's story was featured in the 2013 CNN documentary *Weed*, other families started seeking the treatment, and Charlotte's Web is now sold commercially to help other epileptic children. The oil is also the inspiration behind the Charlotte's Web Medical Access Act, a bill under consideration by Congress that would remove the federal prohibition on marijuana strains that have little or no THC and therefore don't cause users to feel high. *Source: Realm of Caring Foundation, Reset.me, Epilepsy Foundation of Colorado.*

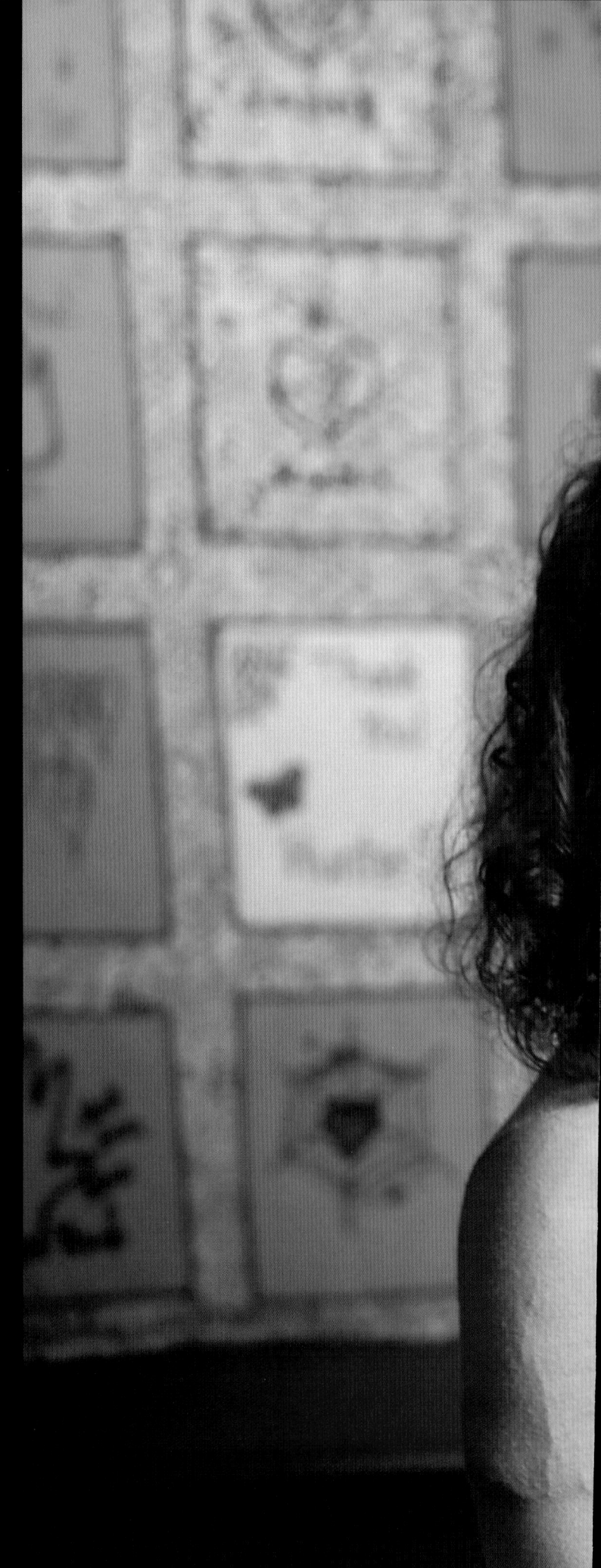

"I WOULD CHALLENGE THEM TO HOLD THEIR CHILD IN THEIR ARMS WHILE THEY ARE NOT BREATHING AND AFTER YOU'VE EXHAUSTED ALL OF YOUR OPTIONS, AND TELL ME WHAT THEY'D DO. IT'S A *PLANT*."

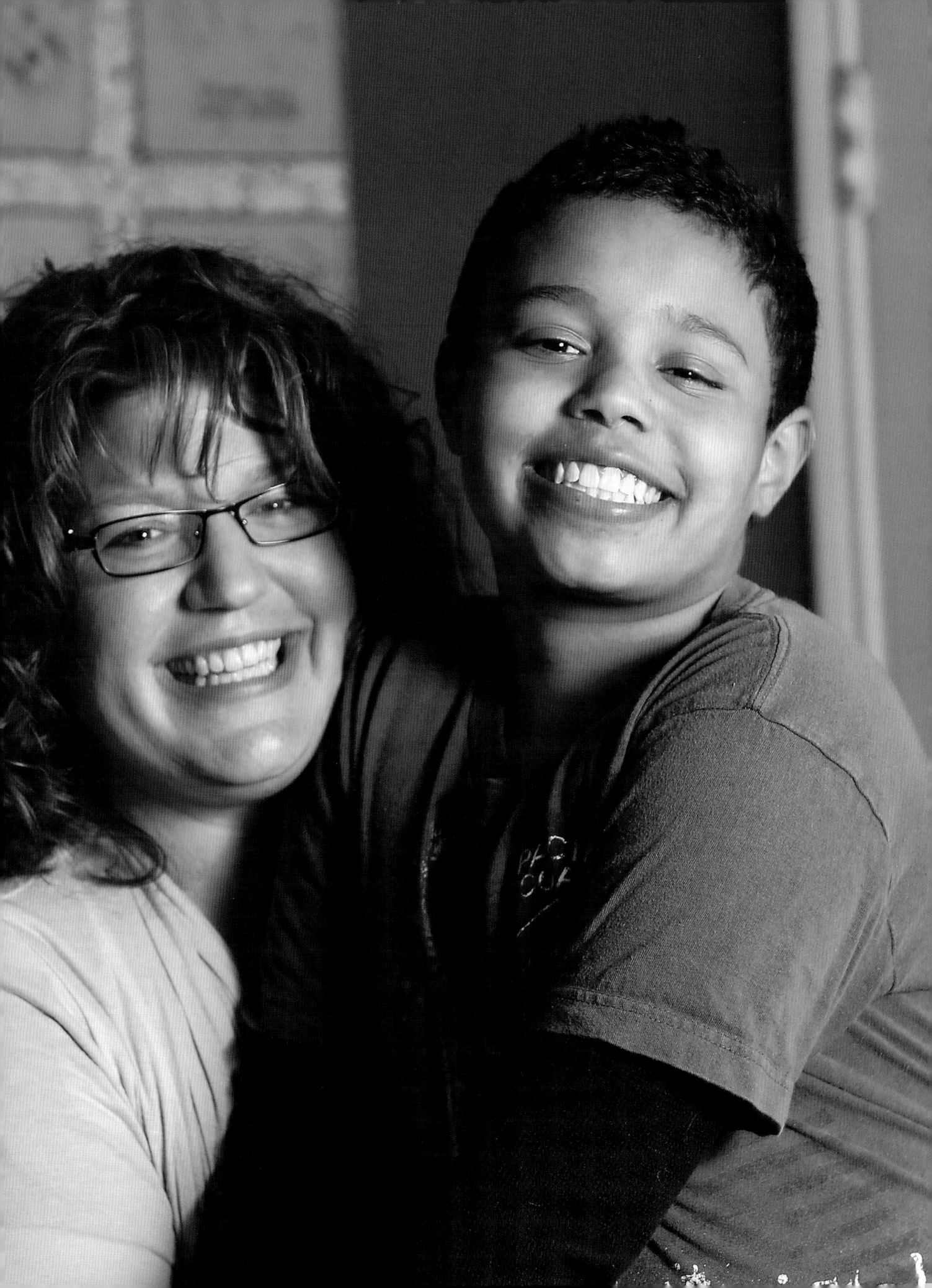

delivered as an egg is ominously cracked into a sizzling frying pan—that informed Heather's views on marijuana. "I thought cannabis can't be good for you, that's for sure," she says, "[that] it kills your brain cells and it's addictive."

As a conservative and a Christian, she was concerned about what her family and friends might think. "Not more concerned, though," she says, "than I was for my son's health. Which is why, after I dug into the research, I accepted that it was an anticonvulsant."

"We didn't have anything to lose at this point," she adds.

It was a fortunate coincidence that the Jackson family lived in Colorado Springs, a mecca of cannabis treatment for pediatric epilepsy. It is just outside of this 440,000-person city that Charlotte's Web is grown, a high-CBD strain that has become particularly popular for addressing epilepsy. Hundreds—400 by Heather's estimation—of other families have fled their home states and flocked to Colorado, particularly Colorado Springs, in a quest for safe, legal access to this medicine. The Jacksons needed to drive just 10 minutes from their home to pick up Zaki's Charlotte's Web.

Heather was still skeptical when, on July 19, 2012, they gave it a try for the first time. Following the nightly bedtime routine of a bath, diaper, and book, she opened the bottle of Charlotte's Web extract, filled the syringe with a low dose of the viscous amber medicine (the for-

mula at the time used honey as the base liquid), and squirted it into his mouth. Then she waited, staring at the time on her phone, counting the minutes as they passed. Suddenly, it was morning—she awoke startled, only to realize that Zaki did not have a seizure all night.

Her hope grew when an unheard of 48 hours passed without a seizure. She slowly raised Zaki's dose over the coming months, and the seizures were sporadic.

Zaki had his last big seizure on Oct. 3, 2012.

"It has literally put his condition into remission," Heather says, speaking just after the 30-month seizure-free mark.

Without seizures standing in his way, Zaki has made leaps and bounds developmentally. Before trying cannabis he was still, in most ways, a toddler: he had to wear pull-up diapers. He didn't know his colors or how to write his name. Today, now 12 years old, he's mastered colors and his name, and is working on the alphabet and numbers. The family is looking for a school for him to attend.

"He's learning concepts he hadn't been able to grasp before," Heather says. "What's even more exciting is the social aspect—he used to have very severe autistic tendencies. Now he has friends and plays and rides a bike. These might be little things to other families, but to us, it's huge. He's living life."

"IT WOULD SET HIM BACK MONTHS DEVELOPMENTALLY AND ALL OF THE HARD WORK WE DID EVERY DAY WAS JUST GONE. I'D CRUMBLE AND GIVE UP AND SCREAM AND YELL AND KICK, AND THEN I'D GET UP IN THE MORNING AND BRUSH MYSELF OFF AND SAY, BECAUSE OF HIM, WE'VE GOTTA CONTINUE ON."

LIFE-CHANGING IMPROVEMENTS

No longer hampered by his suffering, Zaki's spirit has burst forth in full force.

"Zaki is a giggler," his mother begins when asked to describe him. "He's airy. He's got the greatest sense of humor. He's funny. He's very sensitive, very sweet. He's extremely active—like the Energizer Bunny. He's constantly playing, wants to go outside, climb a tree, ride a bike. He's amazing."

The improvements Zaki has made because of cannabis have also been life changing for his parents, who have been together since high school, and his older brother, Zarek, all of whom were also hostages of the condition.

"I just recognized five or six months ago that it wasn't the first thing I did in the morning to go check on Zaki," she says. "His healing is allowing our family to heal. Our schedule doesn't revolve around him and his seizures and whether we can make it to Christmas dinner or not."

Heather didn't rest on her laurels with the morsels of spare time this afforded her. Along with Paige Figi, whose daughter Charlotte was the inspiration and impetus behind the famous Charlotte's

Web strain, Heather started the nonprofit Realm of Caring in 2012 to connect families with information and resources.

She tells Zaki's story, both to the press and through advocacy, in hopes of sparing other families the same extended pain they endured. Although she's since grown a thick skin, Heather says the criticism this can incur is disheartening.

"You do a news [interview] then you read the comments, and people are mean and ignorant and come from a place of misunderstanding," she says. "They have not walked in my shoes. I would challenge them to hold their child in their arms while they are not breathing and after you've exhausted all of your options, and tell me what they'd do. It's a *plant*."

One of her chief goals is to encourage better research in the field, because "as wonderful and healing as Zaki's story is, it's still considered anecdotal evidence." It's time an appropriate amount of funding and research was put into understanding marijuana as medicine, she says.

"This isn't a political issue," she adds. "This is a human rights issue. I want us to stop making political decisions that could literally be life or death for a family."

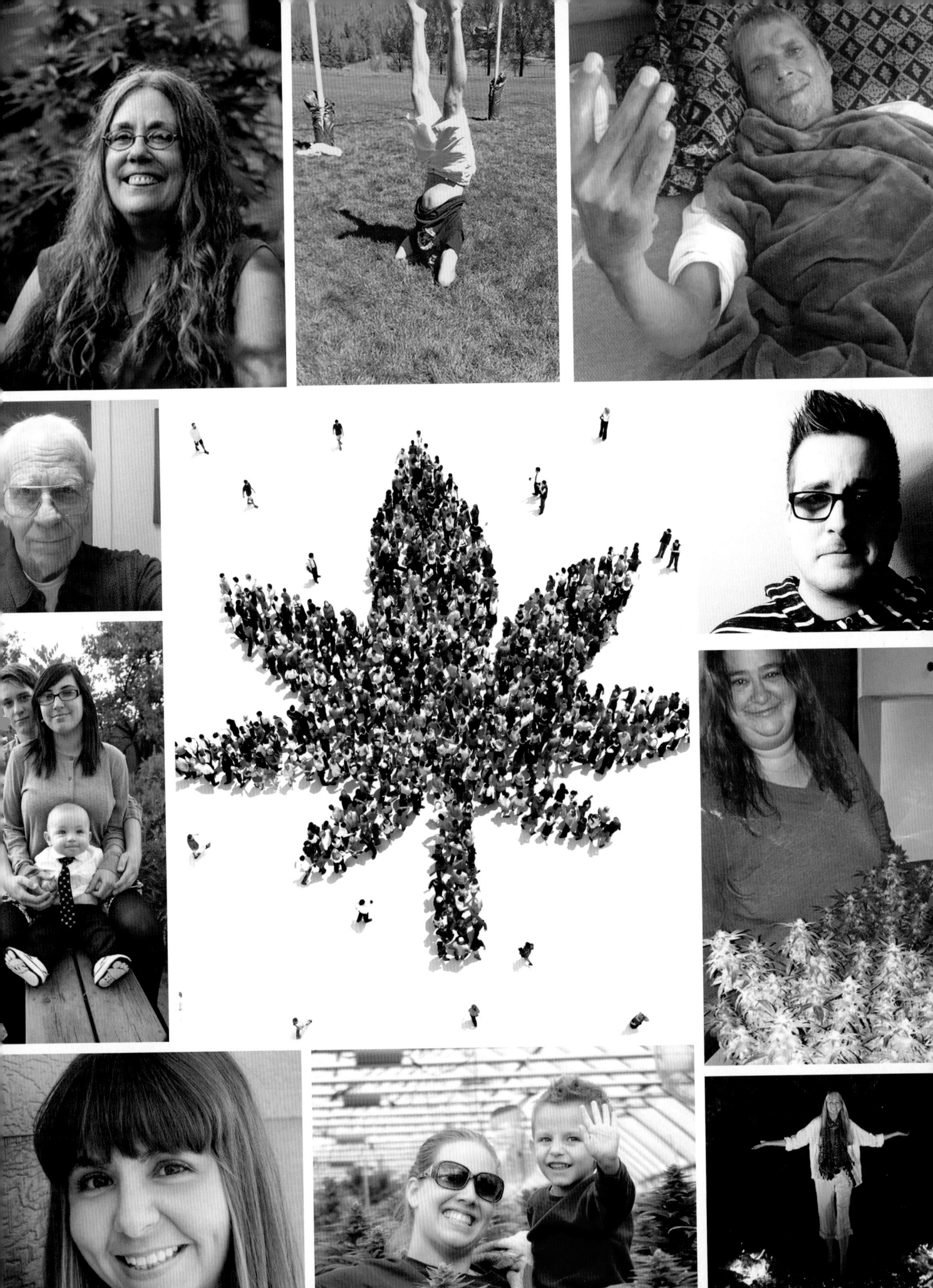

IN
THEIR
OWN
WORDS

FIRST-PERSON ACCOUNTS

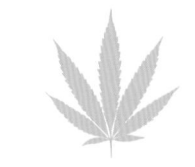

BRANDON BRYANT

Age 39 / **Torn Cornea** / Long Beach, California

Cannabis saved my eyesight. I had an injury in my left eye—a tear in the cornea. It healed but kept tearing at random times, putting me in excruciating pain.

The solution that was offered to me was to burn the surface of my eye off with a laser and let it regrow, which didn't sound good to me. Then I had a doctor suggest cannabis to reduce the pressure of the fluid in my eyes, taking the surface tension off. I started using cannabis and it has never torn since then. Had I not done that, I would have lost my eyesight due to scarring if the cornea kept tearing.

I have 20/20 vision still and no pain for years, thanks to cannabis.

I WOULD HAVE LOST MY EYESIGHT DUE TO SCARRING.

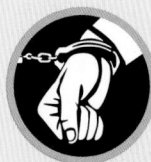

SCHEDULE I: The federal Controlled Substance Act defines Schedule I substances as "drugs with no currently accepted medical use and a high potential for abuse." This listing means that the substances in question are strictly forbidden by federal law, and research on them requires special, difficult-to-acquire permission to perform. Cannabis is categorized as a Schedule I substance despite overwhelming evidence of its numerous medical benefits and no evidence that it is harmful or toxic. As a result, between 1999 and 2014, the federal government approved only 16 independent studies of medical marijuana on humans, according to *Time* magazine.

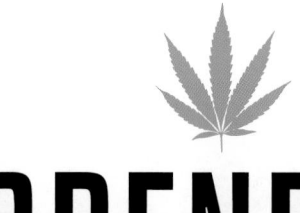

BRENDEN LOZANO

Age 34 / **Depression, Anxiety** / San Diego, California

I witnessed NASA's *Challenger* space shuttle explode while I was on our front lawn in Florida at the age of 4. I was well aware that most passengers on board were ordinary citizens, and this troubled me.

There were many signs of fear and depression early on in my life. For example, I avoided school in fourth grade almost completely, missing more than 100 days that year. I was terrified of leaving my home. But it became unbearable at age 17. Unable to go to school anymore, I dropped out of high school, and society, even though I had been a good student prior to that.

Only recently have I been able to make real progress on my path to waking up my consciousness and beginning to heal. I saw many medical experts and tried every therapy I could find—psychotherapy, medicine, biofeedback, electroshock therapy, hypnotism, and endless other avenues—and all failed in every way.

My hope returned only when I found medical cannabis in California. [At that point] I was ready to move on from Earth.

I consider myself a pretty strong person. I'm not the type to draw attention to myself by threatening to end my life. I never really understood a failed suicide attempt because I always thought, "If I ever got to that point, I would leave no room for error." And although I never attempted suicide, I did come to a point where I was suffering so much anguish that I saw the possibilities in my uni-

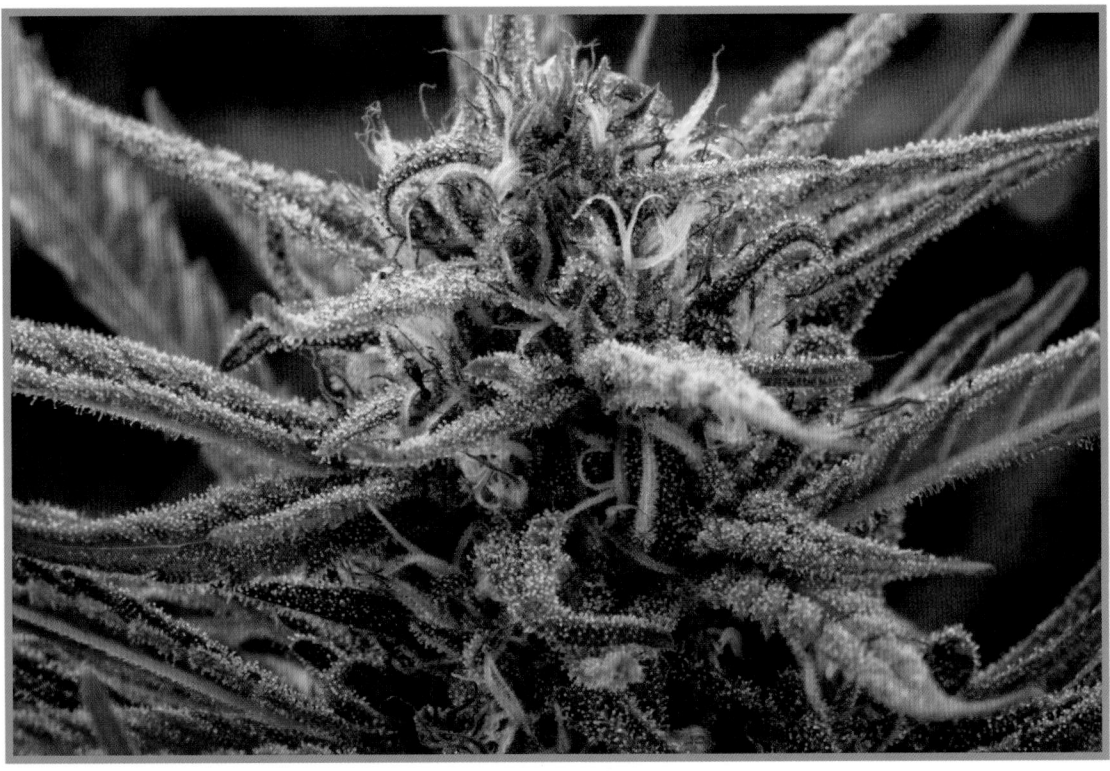

I AVOIDED SCHOOL IN FOURTH GRADE ALMOST COMPLETELY, MISSING MORE THAN 100 DAYS THAT YEAR.

verse shrink to one: suicide. I mean, I really don't understand how people can have depression and still hold a job and carry on with their lives because, in my case at least, I felt the demons devouring me—from the inside out. [It was] other-worldly suffering 24/7. No peace, ever.

Then I remembered about medical cannabis. I got my card immediately and never looked back. I know it saved my life.

For the 17 years I was on many combinations of pills, I did not grow as a person. They stunt your ability to develop naturally. Now that I'm off them, I can't begin to tell you how much more insight I've gained about my condition and the staggering rate my awareness is expanding. Everyone notices. It's like I'm making up for all the lost time. And I'm finally starting to improve notice-ably. I was surprised at how much better I feel physically now that I'm off the medications. It's a huge difference.

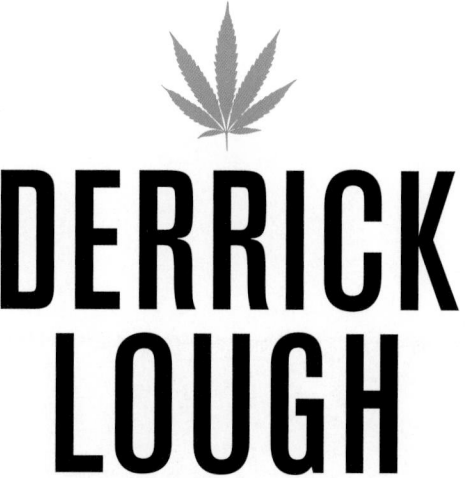

DERRICK LOUGH

Age 30 / **Anxiety** / Denver, Colorado

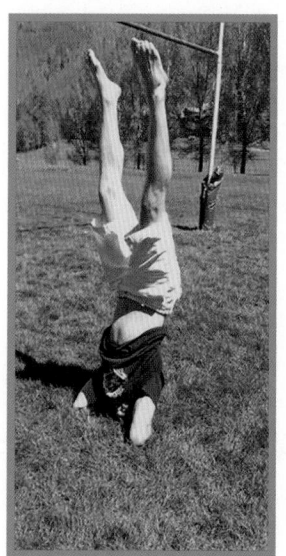

Since childhood I have been dealing with the effects of childhood trauma that came from the abuse by my NPD [Narcissistic Personality Disorder] father.

I listened to many of [spiritual teacher and author] Eckhart Tolle's teachings for years, desperately hoping for peace. Soon after my panic attacks were leaving me bedridden, and I had been taken to my college medical center, at around 28 I started using cannabis for the first time since I was 19. I noticed that with certain activities it would sometimes open a door for letting go of my past pain.

After years of moderately mixing marijuana edibles and yoga, I feel more balanced, compassionate, confident, socially comfortable and at peace.

SINCE I WAS A KID I NEVER THOUGHT I COULD STAND UPSIDE DOWN. IT'S SILLY BUT TRUE. I CAN NOW DO A COUPLE OF UPSIDE-DOWN YOGA POSITIONS.

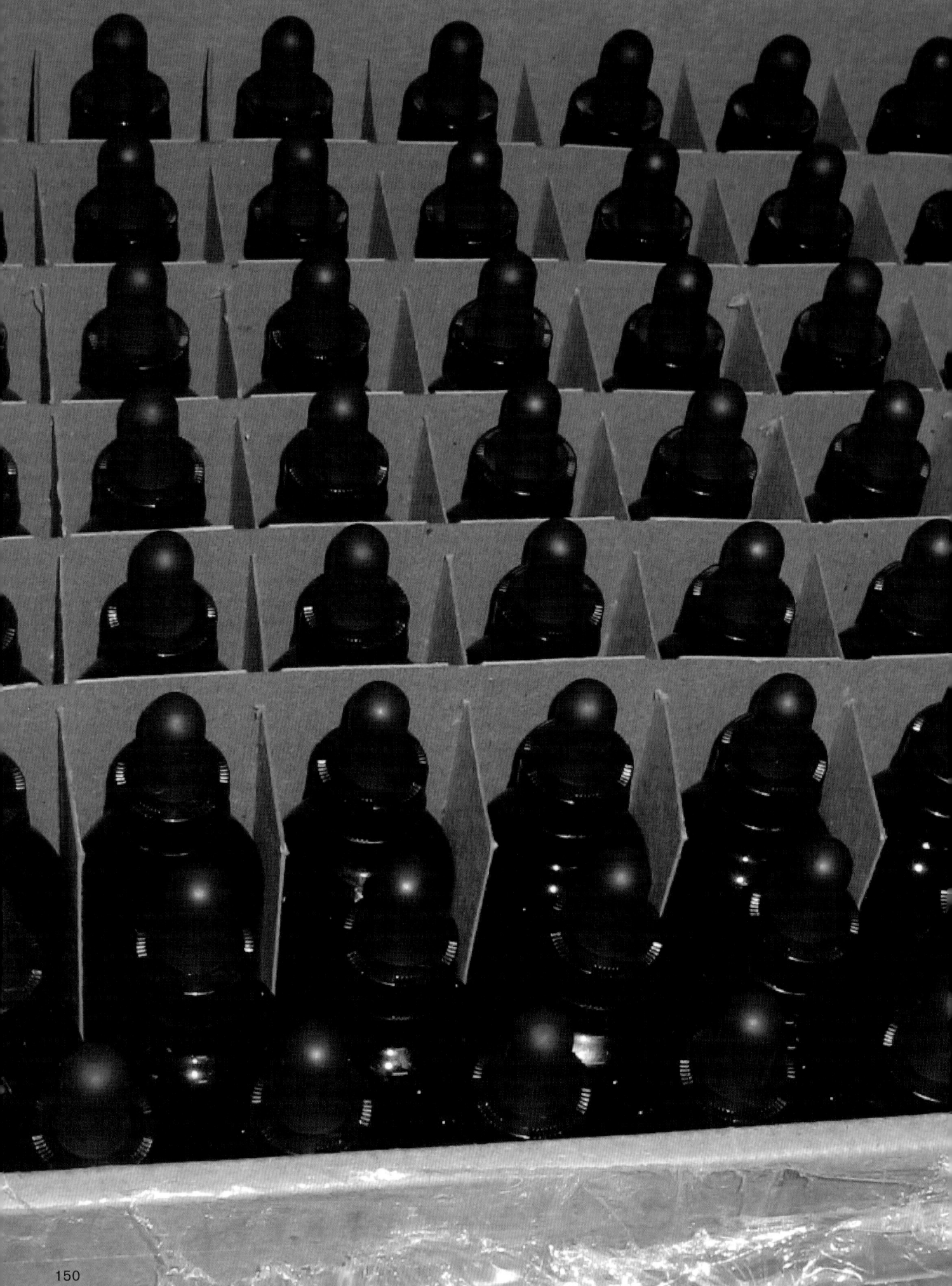

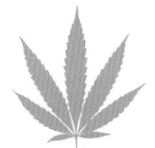

JAMES PROVOST

Age 75 / **Alcohol Dependence, Back Pain, Enlarged Prostate, Gout** / Fair Oaks, California

I have an SB420 license for medical marijuana in California. I am 75 at this time, and have been using it for about four years.

For one year I used 50 percent THC/.8 percent CBD cannabis oil. It reduced my swollen prostate problem by about 80 percent. Then I switched to 70 percent THC/20 percent CBD ("Honey") and it reduced the problem to zero.

I developed gout during the first year. The medication the doctor gave me took about a month to eliminate the pain. It came back before I finished the medication. I used the "Honey" and eliminated it completely.

In the first month using the oil, I lost 25 pounds. [I went from] 200 pounds to 175, and I am now at 172 pounds.

Cannabis is a "thinking drug." Every time I get high I learn something about myself—like [that] the problems in my marriage were small compared to the love.

I started walking 1.25 miles about four times a week. The relaxation and peace I get is amazing.

IN THE FIRST MONTH USING THE OIL, I LOST 25 POUNDS. [I WENT FROM] 200 POUNDS TO 175.

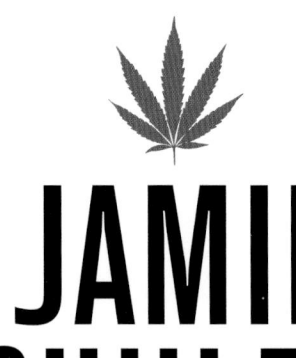

JAMIE SHULER

Age 29 / **Bipolar Disorder** / Los Angeles, California

After being medicated for nearly 10 years for bipolar disorder—and being given every drug under the sun for the first half of that—I decided in early 2014 that I would attempt going off the meds.

I felt very balanced and began to wonder if the meds possibly were holding me back, instead of helping. I still had episodes occasionally, but I wanted to try to go without.

My last dose was Lamictal on June 13, 2014. The first three to four months were very difficult, but one morning, during a particularly hard manic episode, my partner suggested I try smoking a little marijuana to see if it would help calm me down. Before this, I would smoke before bed to help with sleep, or just for relax-ation, but I had never tried it as medicine during a manic episode.

Well, it worked—*really* worked—and I've been using it to curb and control my episodes ever since. I've learned that certain strains of cannabis work better than others, and overall I can honestly say I have never had such amazing results for my mental and emotional health issues.

The best way I can describe it is that, when an episode is happening, everything becomes very fast and out of control. And when I use cannabis during an episode, everything slows down, and I am able to see things with a much clearer perspective. I can usually recover from an episode in about 15 minutes after I smoke, whereas before it would sometimes be hours, or even days.

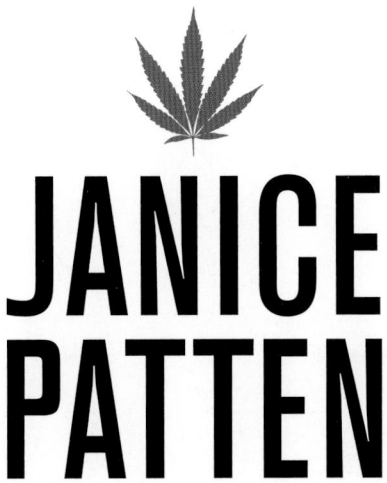

JANICE PATTEN

Age 47 / **Intra-Cranial Hypertension** / Aloha, Oregon

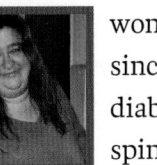

This disease keeps my body from absorbing spinal fluid like everyone else, and causes terrible migraines, blindness and seizures.

The only treatment for it is a medication called Diamox, which causes kidney damage and will eventually shut your kidneys down, along with continued painful spinal taps or a brain surgery that has less than a 20 percent chance of survival—at least that is what doctors will tell you.

I found an article on Rick Simpson Oil and decided to try it—and it works wonders. I have not had a headache since I started the oil. I am no longer diabetic. And I have not had to have a spinal tap, either.

It is apparent to me that cannabis oil is the *only* thing known to man that keeps down spinal fluid. I have not had that surgery, nor am I still taking any of the medications that made me sicker than I was.

I started using this oil in October 2013 and I am alive today because of cannabis—and that is the truth.

I HAVE NOT HAD A HEADACHE SINCE I STARTED THE OIL. I AM NO LONGER DIABETIC.

153

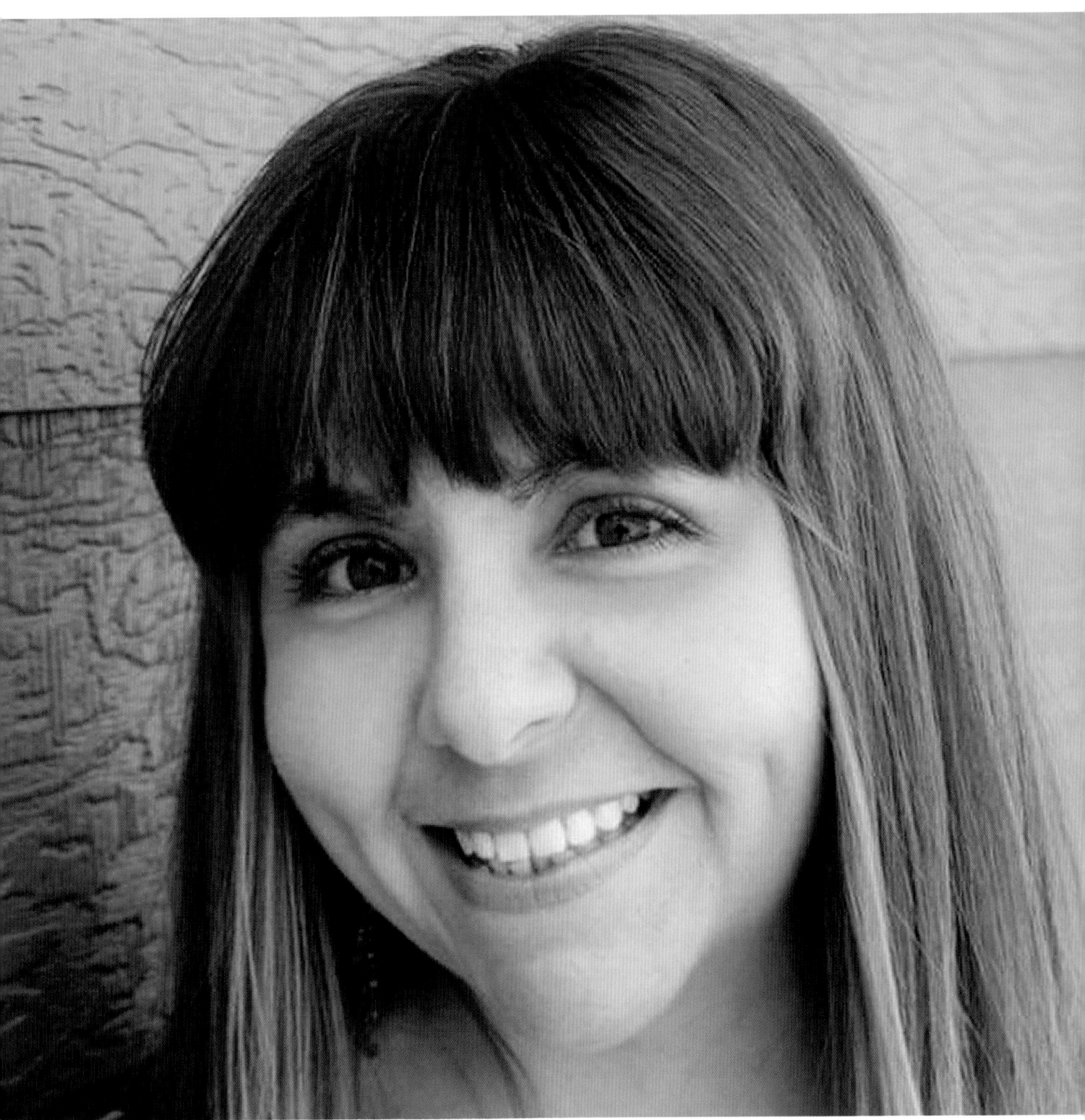

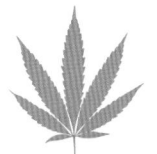

JORDAN PERSON

Age 35 / **Liver Tumor, Kidney Failure, Sepsis, Hysterectomy** / Denver, Colorado

My pain started on my right side just under my rib cage. It was present for a little over a year before it got to the point where I sought medical treatment. They did every test you can imagine, and with each test I received a new pharmaceutical drug, but the only thing that made me feel better was cannabis.

In 2010, the doctors decided to take my gallbladder. When I was in surgery they discovered a tumor on my liver. After seeing a liver specialist I was told the tumor was inoperable and benign, that it was caused by excess estrogen from birth-control pills. I was told I could not have children at that time due to the tumor's location and size.

Every day, post-op, instead of getting

WITHOUT CANNABIS, I WOULD NOT BE HERE. I WOULD HAVE STAYED ON ALL THE PILLS AS PRESCRIBED AND WOULD HAVE PROBABLY DIED FROM SEPTICEMIA. I CAN SAY WITH PRIDE THAT CANNABIS SAVED MY LIFE.

I REFUSED THE PAINKILLERS AND USED CANNABIS FOR EVERY SYMPTOM I HAD.

better, I got worse, until eventually my skin began turning yellowish gray. I called my mom in Colorado and told her I felt like I was dying. I left Florida the next day, leaving my dog, car and everything I owned.

On my second day in Colorado, I received my medical marijuana card, but two weeks later I ended up in the ER being prepped for emergency surgery. They discovered a 9mm stone in my right kidney that had put me into sepsis. My blood was toxic and my kidneys were shutting down. Two surgeries later they were able to remove the stone. However, I refused the painkillers and used cannabis for every symptom I had. The nausea, the anxiety, and the pain were all treated by the same plant instead of the numerous pharmaceuticals they wanted me to take.

The pain continued and moved lower into my body, and it resulted in a total abdominal hysterectomy in 2011. The recovery from surgery was unbearable. I ingested more cannabis than I can

describe. Four weeks post-op they discovered they made an error while suturing me closed and my ureter had been occluded. I was in kidney failure once again. I was prepped for another emergency surgery, this time to insert a nephrostomy tube. The tube drained urine from my kidney to a bag on my thigh for six and a half months until they could go in and fix things with a non-refluxing ureteral implantation. This gave me a new ureter on my bladder.

My final surgery came when a surgeon at the Porter Hospital for Liver Care got a hold of my chart and wanted to see me. I ended up having the "inoperable" tumor removed on Dec. 12, 2012, thus closing the three-year, six-surgery cycle of my life.

Without cannabis, I would not be here. I would have stayed on all the pills as prescribed and would have probably died from septicemia. I can say with pride that cannabis saved my life.

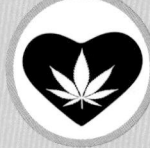

COMPASSIONATE USE: Compassionate use is when a drug or treatment that has not been approved by the U.S. Food and Drug Administration is used with permission, outside of official clinical trials. A small handful of patients were permitted to use, and were supplied with, cannabis by the federal government starting in the 1970s after patient Robert Randall successfully argued in court that he needed marijuana to control his glaucoma. The compassionate investigational new drug program for marijuana was closed to new patients in 1992, and today only four people still receive cannabis from the government. *Source: U.S. Food and Drug Administration, medicalcannabis.com.*

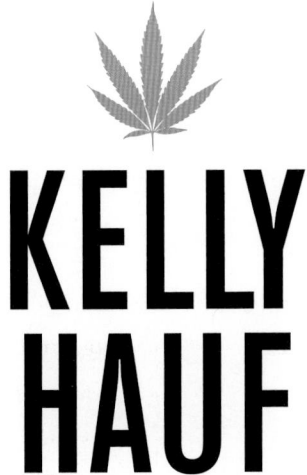

KELLY HAUF

Age 53 / **Brain Tumor** / Tuolumne, California

I was diagnosed with a 3-centimeter brain tumor in my left frontal lobe in January 2000.

I had a craniotomy in September 2003, in which the surgeon felt confident that all visible tumor had been removed. No chemotherapy or radiation was recommended at that time. I have been monitored via MRI of the brain every three to six months since diagnosis. I've had well over 50 MRIs to date. In November 2013, my MRI revealed that the tumor was growing back.

After doing a lot of research, I decided to try cannabis oil instead of the recommended chemotherapy. My husband retired as an assistant chief at the fire department, we sold our house in Oklahoma, and we moved to San Francisco to do my treatment where it was legal. After eight months total of cannabis-concentrated oil treatment, the MRI revealed that only scar tissue remained. I've had one other MRI to date, which also shows no tumor growth present. Not only did the cannabis kill the brain tumor cells, but it also took away all my lower back and shoulder pain during my treatment.

I would like others to consider this healthier option of treatment for their tumors and cancers before trying the more aggressive and harsh treatments that can do more harm in the long term.

I would also like others to know that it is doable to move out of state to seek cannabis treatment in a legal state if yours does not allow it. It is not easy to pick up and move, but it's worth it to save your life, or a loved one's life.

EDITOR'S NOTE: FOR MORE ON KELLY'S STORY, PLEASE VISIT: KELLYSHEALINGPATH.COM.

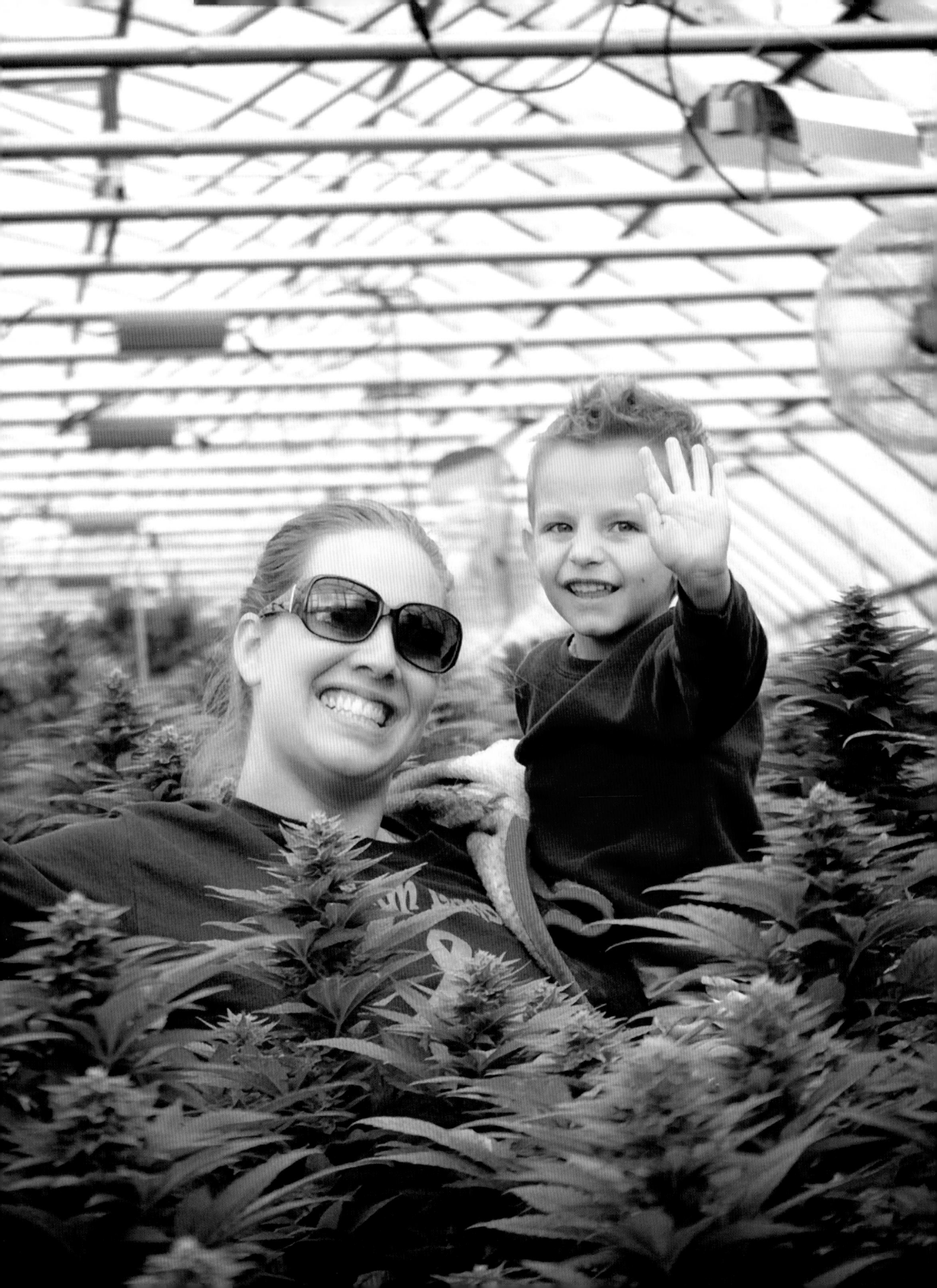

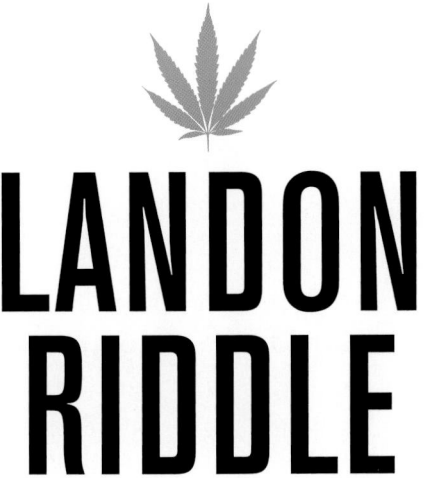

LANDON RIDDLE

Age 5 / **Leukemia** / Colorado Springs, Colorado

As told by Landon's mother, Sierra Riddle, from a post that originally appeared on teamlandon-cannabis.blogspot.com.

In our craze of researching for something to keep my son Landon alive during chemotherapy for his Leukemia, we came across many studies that showed cannabis could give him a good quality of life while fighting the cancer, and give him the relief the narcotics and pharmaceuticals couldn't give him.

Landon, then 2 years old, started taking cannabis in January 2013. Soon after his first dose of cannabis, he was feeling a lot better than he had in months. People always ask me if it was hard to convince the two doctors to recommend Landon for the medical marijuana program. Those doctors took one look at Landon and his cancer file and signed for his red card. They could see just how ill he was, as could everyone else.

We were still living in Utah and going through intense chemo treatment, so my mother, Landon and I started a very grueling dual residency [in Colorado] in order to get Landon's cannabis treatments, as they were showing us the first glimpses of hope. He started getting better and better. As the weeks went on, the chemo's side effects seemed to lessen and lessen. His severe neuropathy, caused directly by one of the chemotherapies, was healing itself. His reflexes started regenerating and his vomiting decreased to 10 times per day or less. He was up and awake most of the day now, walking a little, laughing and trying to be as normal as possible.

I think the most important and the most miraculous thing was that Landon started to enjoy life again. He was finally able to do more than sit on our couch or in bed and vomit for weeks on end. He was finally able to eat, enjoy it and keep it down. Cannabis was starting to give him back what chemo had stolen!

Landon was now doing amazingly, and his doctors in Utah could not figure out why, especially since he had done so badly with the chemo for so long. The cannabis was doing far more for Landon than just helping with his pain and nausea. It was helping Landon on a cellular level, as well. The weekly blood results were showing us in black and white the powers of cannabis. The amount of blood and platelet transfusions needed after chemo was cut by 75 percent, and he no longer needed the IV promethazine or morphine. In fact, Landon no longer needed any pharmaceuticals for pain, nausea, anxiety, sleep, or night terrors. Cannabis took the place of around a dozen or more medications filling my cabinet. His immune system was kept high and he no longer caught every virus that floated by in the air.

He was able to enjoy time with family and explore things again. He was now getting stronger every day, able to walk distances he hadn't in many months, and strong enough to walk up and down the stairs again with minimal assistance. He was able to go out in the sunshine without fear of chemo rash. I am still amazed as I sit here writing this that one little old plant saved my son's life.

Finally it seemed we were done with intense chemo and headed into maintenance—the longest, but supposedly easiest, course of chemo in the Leukemia roadmap. This round also included steroids five days out of the month. It only took one month of the steroids for us to really question if the side effects of them were worth it, especially considering the long-term aspect. They made Landon very violent and angry, his legs were so swollen you could not see his knees or ankles, and he could not walk again. Could we really justify putting him through this every month for the next three years? Given all we had seen and learned about cannabis, we believe that using only it will keep Landon in remission. I made the choice to end chemo, move to Colorado full time and give cannabis a try solo with no chemo or steroids. The results seen in Landon were mind blowing.

I thought that with it being Colorado, the oncologist would be more supportive of natural cancer treatments. I was very wrong! They do not see anything but chemo as a proven treatment for cancer, and they proceeded to turn my life upside down with [Child Protective Services] reports of medical abuse and meetings with lawyers, etc., all in order to make me comply with their chemo plan for Landon. I had no choice but to comply and allow them to start poisoning my son again—this time for three years.

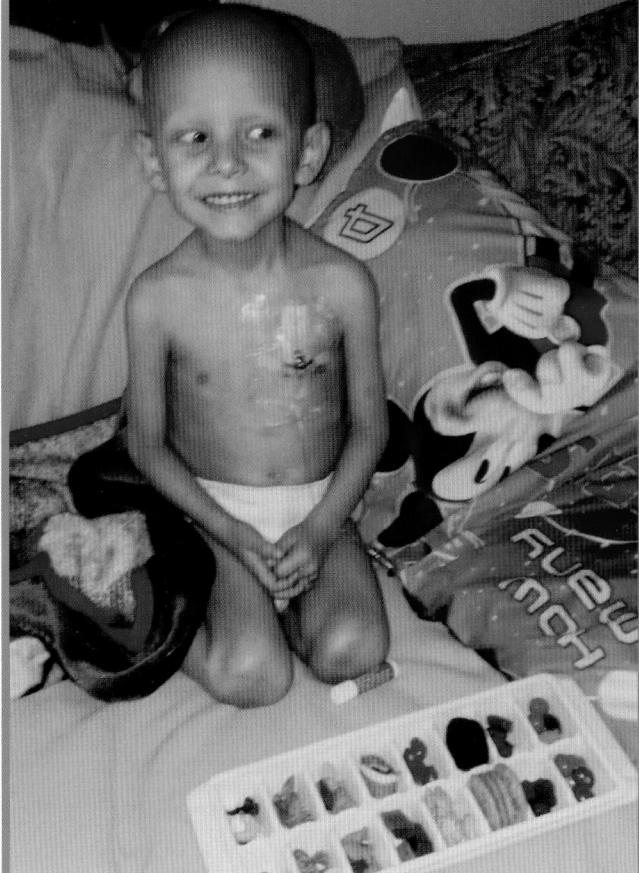

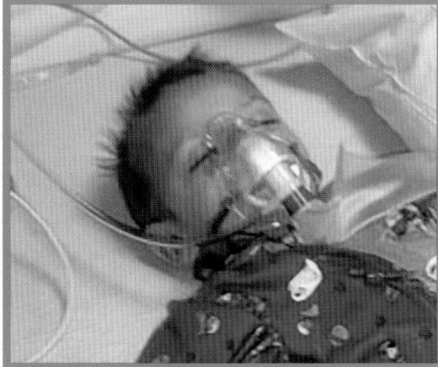

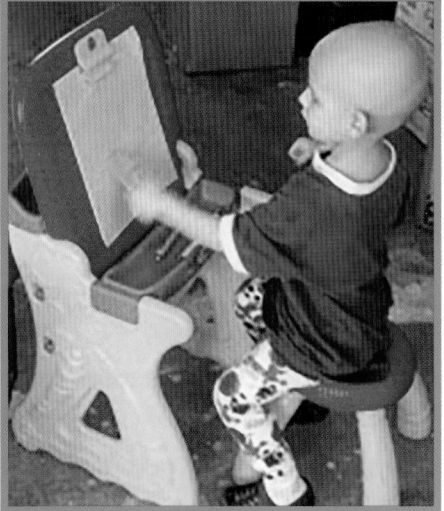

HIS SEVERE NEUROPATHY, CAUSED DIRECTLY BY ONE OF THE CHEMOTHERAPIES, WAS HEALING ITSELF.

We were told this round of chemo would not harm Landon, but we did not see this to be true, sadly. Chemo is toxic to the body and caused burns to Landon's bum, and the effects on his mental and emotional state were devastating.

I will keep trying to spread Landon's story to every corner of the world. I fight for all the Landons in the world right now, at this very moment, who are fighting cancer and for their lives. Team Landon (teamlandon.org) has fought with me every step of the way and will continue to do so. What doctors are doing to a cancer-free 5-year-old is terribly wrong. Our kids deserve a better way, and they don't deserve to suffer aimlessly when cannabis is being grown in many states.

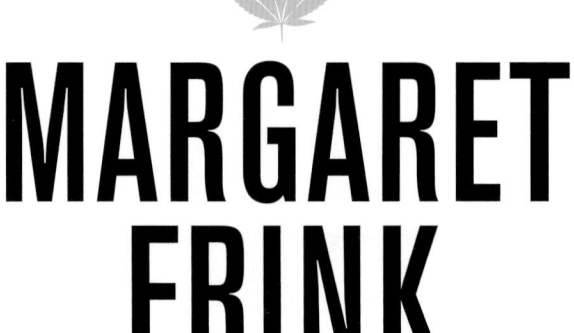

MARGARET FRINK

Age 54 / **Hereditary Neuralgic Amyotrophy** / Portland, Oregon

I'm from a small, almost nonexistent place in North Carolina called Pompey's Ridge, near Smith's Crossing. I grew up on a farm—we had hogs, tobacco and chickens.

We don't have a firm diagnosis, but I saw at least 13 people in my family suffer seriously from this disease, leading to their demise. Two died in my house. I was diagnosed when I was 43. I'm 54 now. We knew we had a serious problem, but we just didn't know what it was. It was a really rare disease. I had a lot of specialized testing before they figured out that it was hereditary neuralgic amyotrophy, a genetic condition that leads to severe intractable pain. They used to call it atypical MS. They had a different name for it every time someone from our family went to the hospital. It's only since the advent of genetic testing that we've been able to learn what's going on in our family.

I tried muscle relaxants, opiates, and acupuncture. I tried some of everything. My quality of life was absolutely miserable. But then an intern at the Cleveland Clinic who was chatting with me mentioned cannabis. So I started reading up on it and it sounded very promising.

Cannabis has made my symptoms much better. I've gotten increased muscle mass. I've gotten off all the other drugs—I'm now just on cannabis and Propanol. My side effects are minimal.

I own a farm in southeast North Carolina, but I can't risk being arrested and losing my property. The worry and fear of using cannabis in a place where it's illegal was too much to bear, so I left for Portland, Oregon, in 2010. I still own the

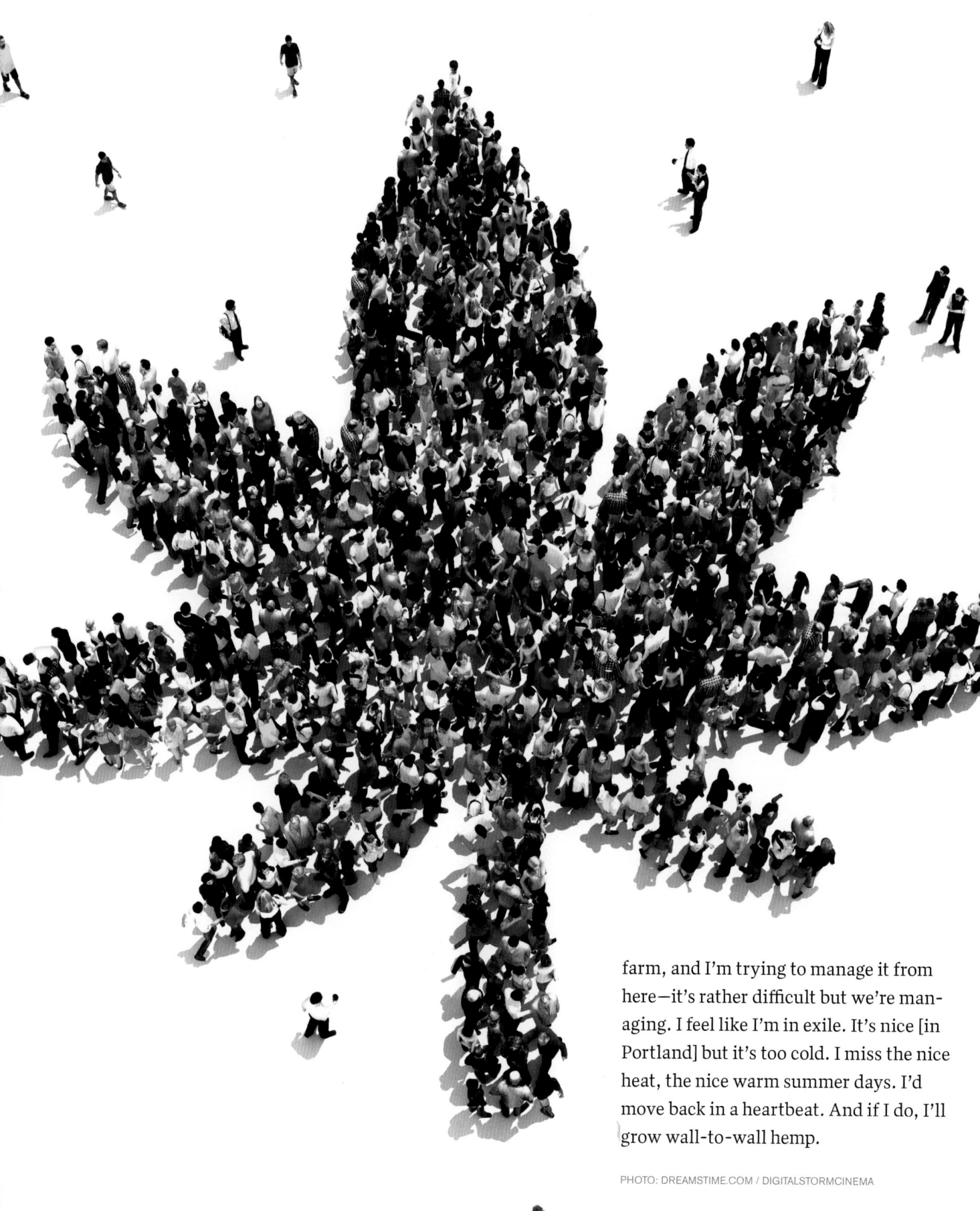

farm, and I'm trying to manage it from here—it's rather difficult but we're managing. I feel like I'm in exile. It's nice [in Portland] but it's too cold. I miss the nice heat, the nice warm summer days. I'd move back in a heartbeat. And if I do, I'll grow wall-to-wall hemp.

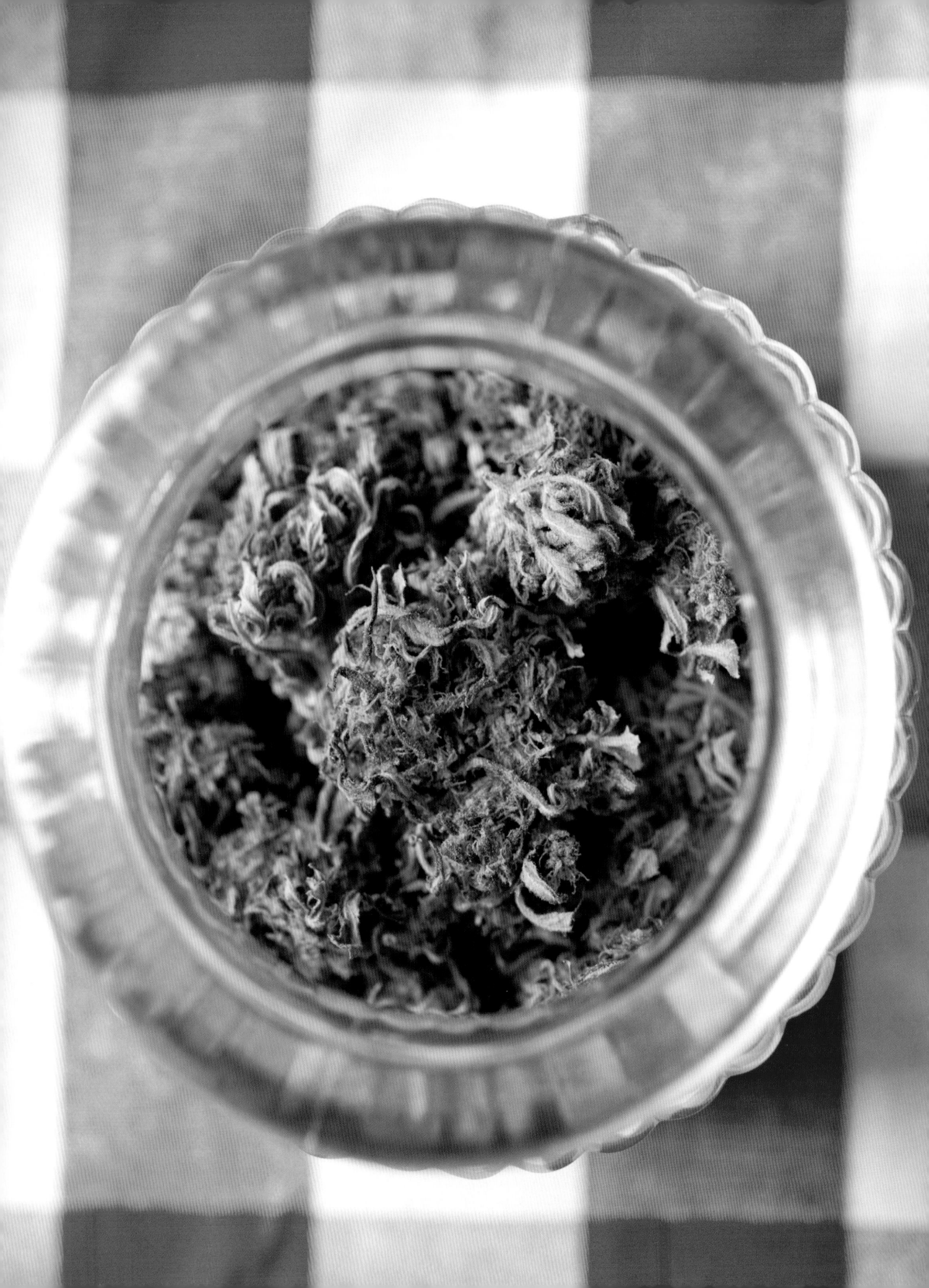

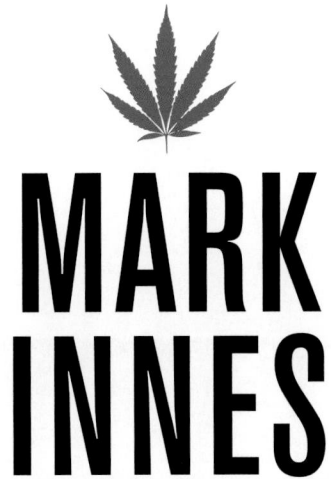

MARK INNES

Age 54 / **Asbestos Poisoning** / Manhattan, Kansas

Asbestos is a fiber with little hooks in it. Because of those hooks, it doesn't allow you to clean it out of your lungs like the other things you breathe in. It makes the inside of your lungs hard—the transference of oxygen isn't as efficient.

When I was diagnosed with asbestos poisoning, doctors wanted me do everything, from taking very potent painkillers to having surgery. They wanted to cut chunks out of me. I said no to everything.

When I was looking into how I could treat myself, I found that if you take the cannabis plant's root, pulverize it and put it in a press to squeeze the oil out of it, you get a very good concentration of cannabidiol (CBD)—a specific cannabinoid that can manage your pain without you getting loopy. When you take pain medications, like hydrocodone, you get loopy. I have a wife, Genny, six kids and many responsibilities, so I didn't want to be loopy. With CBD oil, I was able to stay productive, stay employed, stay happy, to remain in a balance of homeostasis—it's amazing how much your blood pressure is affected when you have chronic pain.

The oil wasn't hard to make; it just wasn't legal. I found the information in the public library, but I couldn't even talk to my doctor about it. So I keep it 100 percent private. It's not a social thing, it's a medicine for me, but I'd love to have help from a medical professional.

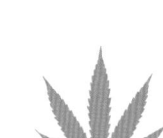

MELANIE BARNISKIS

Age 59 / **Diabetes, Neuropathy, Gout, Breast Cancer** / Phoenix, Oregon

In 2008, I was the 911 supervisor for the city of Bethel, Alaska. When on duty, I was the only 911 operator in an area the size of the state of Oregon. There are no roads to Bethel. Everything comes in and goes out via air, making Bethel the third-busiest airport in Alaska. Large equipment can be brought up by barge during June, July or August, but the costs are astronomical. So the medical assistance available out there is limited—no x-ray machines, CT scanners, MRI machines, etc. Any ailment needing a high level of care has to be done in Anchorage, an hour's flight away.

My insurance company saw no need to authorize $13,000 worth of medevac for me, so the one and only physical therapist in Bethel would pick at my open, diabetic, ulcerated, neuropathic feet with clean tweezers—after handing me some clean paper towels to bite down on when the pain got too bad. This went on weekly for over a year.

Pain relief was impossible. They would not authorize more than 20 to 25mg of Vicodin every two weeks. That means a pill and a half each day, most days. I saved that to try and sleep between shifts at work. The rest of the time I ate 32 to 36 Advil caplets each day: 250mg caplets that I would order by the 500-count bottle, four bottles a month, and no one questioned a thing.

I finally collapsed at work, was taken to the emergency room and determined to be so low in potassium that none registered in blood tests. I spent four hours shivering in the ER and then was sent home with the instructions: "Potassium regulates the heartbeat, and you don't have any. So if your chest hurts, come right back because you are having a heart attack."

It took us 10 months to get out of Bethel. We chose to move to Oregon. After four months here, I tried—or, rather, rediscovered—cannabis. The pain relief was immediate, convincing and literally life changing. In one night I went from a suffering, half-dead, soon-to-be-all-the-way-dead police dispatcher to being a criminal whose feet didn't hurt anymore.

The criminal phase only had to last long enough for me to register with the state of Oregon after submitting my medical reports from Alaska. I qualified under Oregon's medical marijuana program in May 2009. At that time, I was close to 300 pounds. My top recorded weight in Alaska was 347 pounds. I had type-2 diabetes, neuropathy, gout, high blood pressure, bad cholesterol and inflammatory "outbreaks" in numerous joints intermittently.

By 2011, I had lost 40 pounds, had eliminated gout flares and many of the joint flare-ups, and was still taking Lisinopril and Metformin but had developed a cannabis regime that was providing excellent pain relief from the neuropathy. I was even looking forward to having a vegetable garden—something I could not do in Alaska, or anywhere else at 300-plus pounds.

Then I discovered Rick Simpson Oil, the cannabis concentrate, and I began using 400mg daily of my own home-made extract in March 2013. As of now, over two years later, I am off all prescription meds. I have been called a rock star at the doctor's office. My blood pressure is solidly normal and I maintain a regular weight between 150 and 160 pounds through just doing normal things. I ride a bike, walk, garden, and operate in all ways like a fully functional 59-year-old woman—with one difference.

In July 2014, I was diagnosed with Stage 1 breast cancer. I am using only cannabis extract to treat the cancer. I take about 1,200mg a day of THC, and whatever other cannabinoids, terpenes and flavonoids exist in the mix. So far, the medical team around me is documenting and testing but otherwise not doing anything other than shaking their heads and muttering things like "I wish you would agree to the excisional biopsy." But that's not happening.

I have had, seen, felt and experienced such marvelous and impossible—at least with traditional medicine—results from the cannabis that there is no doubt whatsoever that it will cure my cancer. I am literally betting my life on this, and happy to do so.

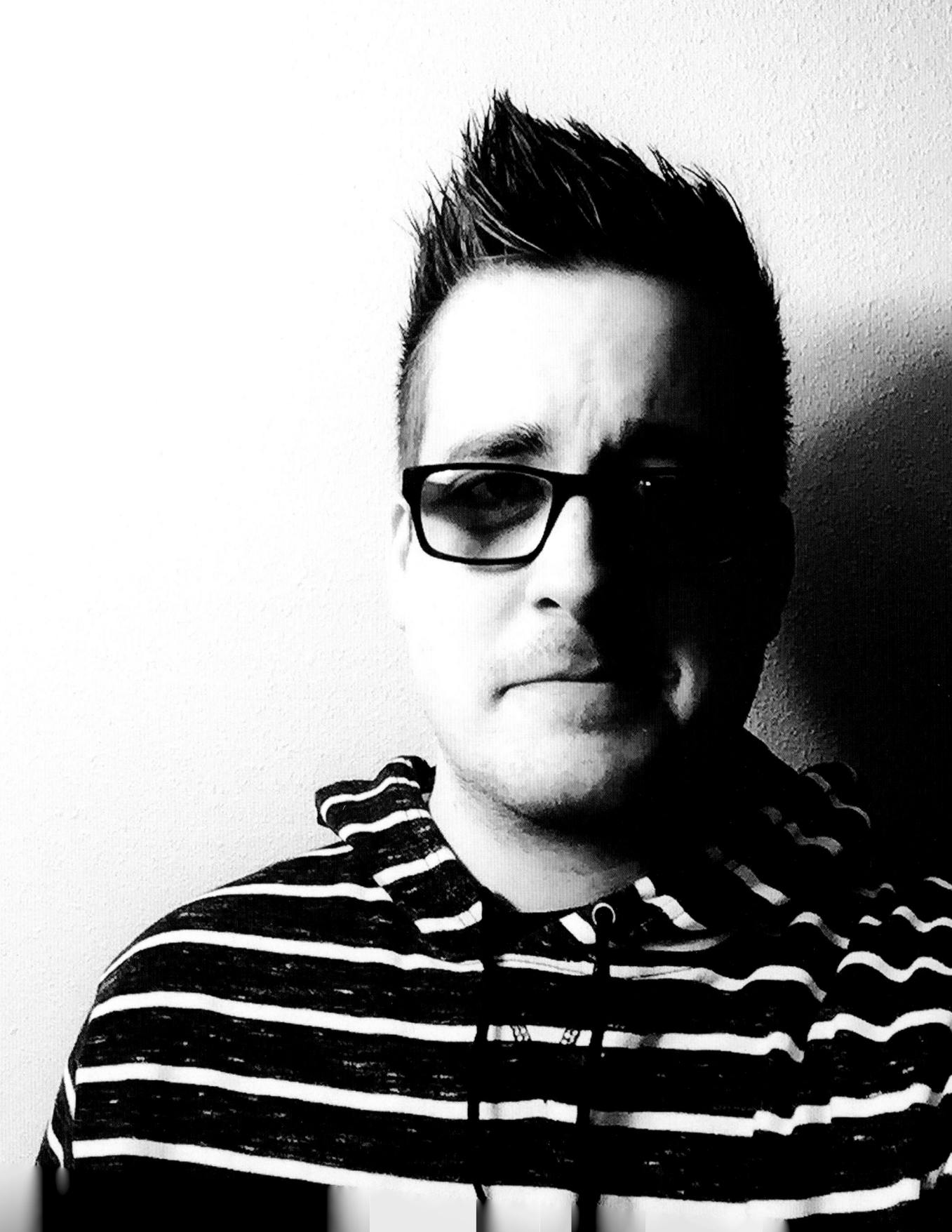

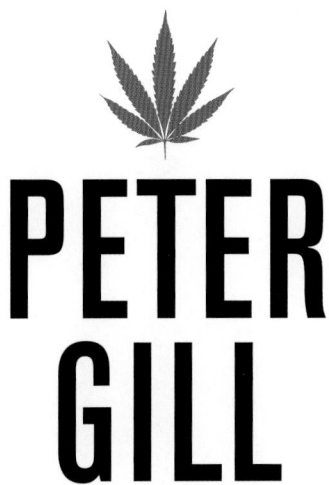

PETER GILL

Age 23 / **Depression** / Portland, Oregon

Three years ago, I was at an all-time low in my life. I was a doubting evangelical Christian who knew that my grand departure from the faith was looming. I struggled to sleep, feel, and engage with living. I had quit my last job and found myself deeply depressed and aimless. I would wake up having panic attacks from dreams of suicide. I would secretly plead with the universe to give me reason again. I desperately needed peace.

A good friend of mine had told me about his cannabis use and invited me to come over and try it with him. I had always been a straight-laced sort of dude, but I found myself desperate. I needed help.

My friend invited me again to try cannabis with him. I decided that it was worth a shot … I immediately felt its effects. We sat down in silence. I found myself at peace with my day and enjoying our time. That night I slept a solid eight hours and woke up wondering why I had not tried this before. Unfortunately, I had to stay clean, because I was still looking for a job.

Fast-forward a few months later, I had the opportunity to move up near Portland, Oregon. I got a great job and found my footing in life again. [Eventually] I became a regular user. From that point on, I found myself sleeping well every single night and not having nightmares. I have new energy and motivation. It has become a daily ritual and meditation. It is my great equalizer.

I am a "hypocrite" to some people who know that I smoke now. I've

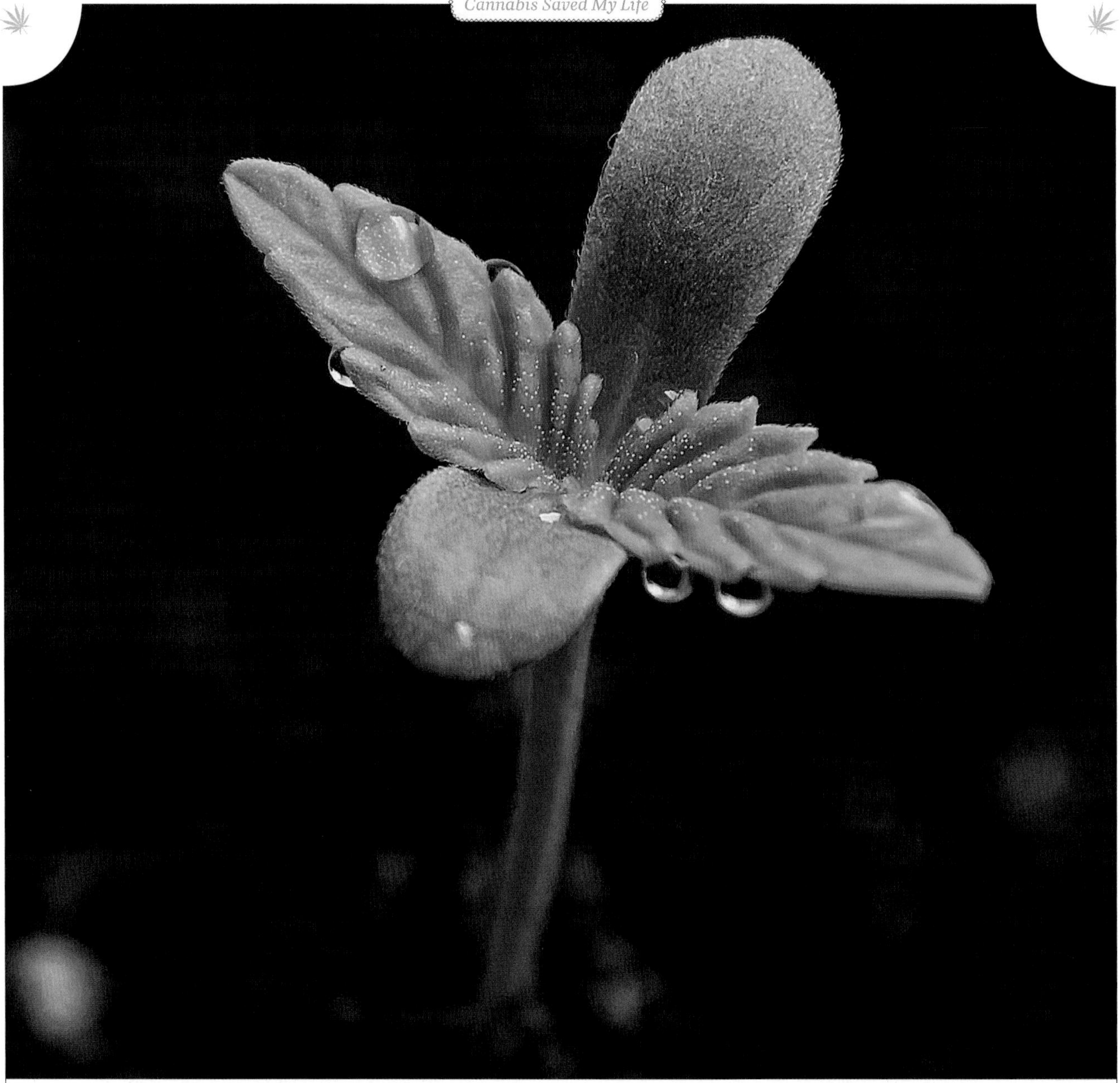

I WOULD WAKE UP HAVING PANIC ATTACKS FROM DREAMS OF SUICIDE. I WOULD SECRETLY PLEAD WITH THE UNIVERSE TO GIVE ME REASON AGAIN. I DESPERATELY NEEDED PEACE.

learned that being wrong about something can be right. I'm OK with my changes and departures. Life is good.

I'm excited to see where legalization goes in America and the world. People need help, and people need peace.

PHOTO: SHUTTERSTOCK / MARIE NIMRICHTEROVA.

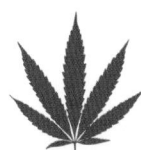

RAMDIAL SINGH SANGHA

Age 64 / Heart Disease, Liver Disease, Neurological Complications, Type 2 Diabetes / San Jose, California

As told by his son, 21-year-old Akashpreet Singh.

My father, Ramdial Singh Sangha, resides in San Jose, California, where he has established a reputation as an honorable, humble man from the people who have been fortunate enough to have him be a part of their life.

Unfortunately, the past few years have been hard for him. Along with medical conditions, he has been going through a lot of emotional distress and started to resort to alcohol to give him relief. Over time, alcohol took over his life. But he fought it, and to my surprise, had successfully gone sober. In 2014, after being sober for a year, he suffered a cirrhotic liver failure that changed his life forever.

Over the years my father has contracted numerous conditions that have hindered his ability to do normal daily activities, so much so that he has started to physically deteriorate. He's been diagnosed with ESLD (end-stage liver disease) with an advanced case of cirrhosis, he has

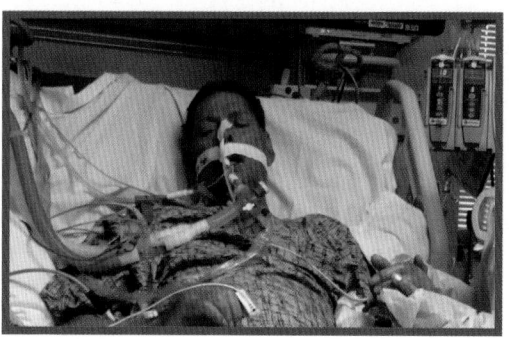

heart disease, he is a Type 2 diabetic, and he has neurological complications as a result of a brain tumor in the late 1990s. His family has a history of cardiac arrest and he himself has undergone two open-heart surgeries in which a total of four stents were placed on his heart.

Mind you, all of these illnesses were diagnosed years before he had a cirrhotic liver failure. Post-liver failure, he was hospitalized for the course of about 11 months. During that stay he became a different person. He went from being totally independent to not being able to walk or stand, not being able to eat, not being able to breath without the help of a ventilator, and not being able to talk or communicate. Even using good judgment to make simple decisions had become an obstacle for him. Every day he progressively grew sicker and sicker to the point where I had convinced myself my father would soon lose his life.

After the hospital stay he had finally come home to what he thought would be normal life, but that wasn't the case. For weeks I followed a strict routine designed for him by highly praised medical professionals who claimed he would never recover to the extent he has. Every day he took more than 20 pills, and was taking five insulin injections daily (his blood sugar averaged 250-350 mg/dL).

At this point, he was starting to lose hope. After seeing enough, I did the unthinkable: against medical advice and behind my family's back, I gave him

Rick Simpson Hemp Oil. One drop and he was a brand-new person. For the first time in a year, I saw him smile. I will never forget that day—he stood up like he had never been sick. It was amazing. I was speechless.

Now, he's gone from 20-plus pills a day to less than 10. His blood sugar is finally stable—he's still insulin-dependent but his blood sugar now averages 120 mg/dL and we've drastically reduced his insulin dosages. Now he can eat without throwing up right away and he doesn't have anxiety attacks. He is finally starting to recover. I never thought I would see him like that again. He is happy again.

Unfortunately I've come to find that cirrhosis is a very dangerous, deadly disease, and it is not an easy fight. He is starting to succumb to the disease again. That being said, I am confident in his efforts to recover and know that cannabis' efficiency as a medicine will make every day easier for him. Cannabis has done for my dad in one week what a whole team of medical professionals couldn't do over six months.

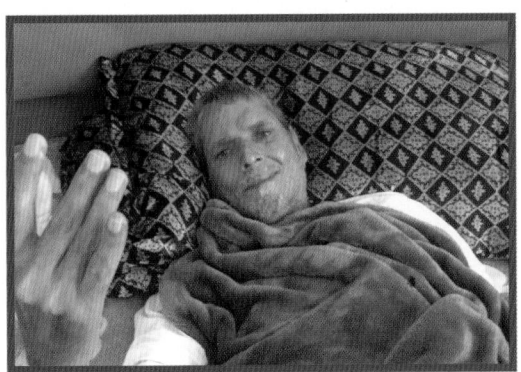

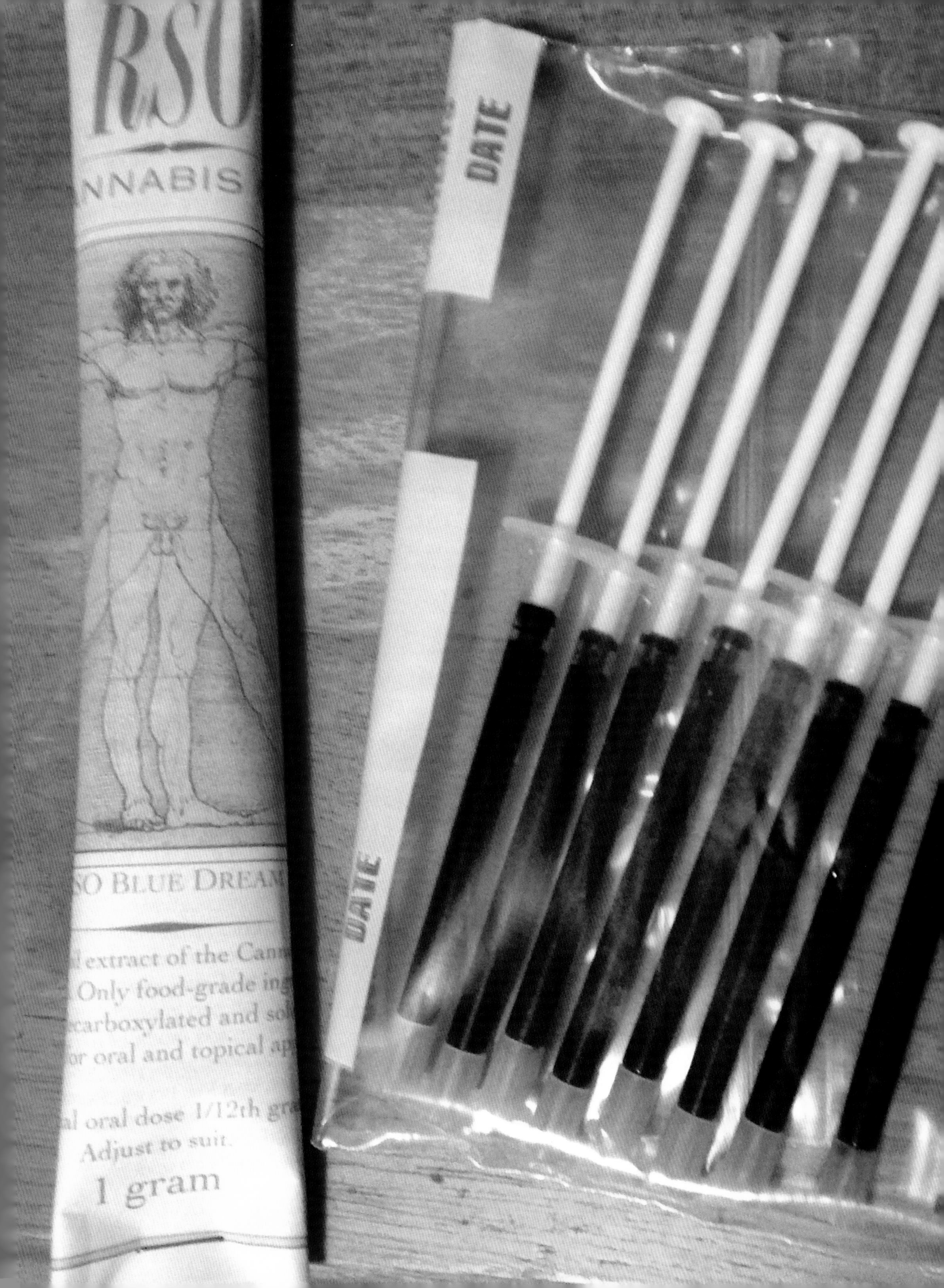

RSO

CANNABIS

SO BLUE DREAM

l extract of the Cann
Only food-grade ing
carboxylated and sol
or oral and topical ap

al oral dose 1/12th gra
Adjust to suit.

1 gram

DATE

DATE

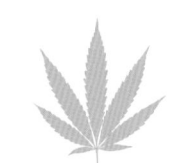

SARAH LAURENT*

Age 37 / **PTSD** / Chicago, Illinois

I was sexually and emotionally abused as a child, and I have PTSD.

I have had a long and painful history of different therapists and doctors. I've taken nine different prescription medications for anxiety and depression. None of the drugs helped. The side effects would be terrible, or they would actually exacerbate my issues or turn me into a zombie.

Then on a trip to Colorado, I ate my first-ever edible—figuring "when in Rome"—and discovered, much to my shock, that I handled several major PTSD triggers that day with far less emotional fallout than usual.

A year ago, I would have told you that the idea that there are legitimate medical applications for cannabis was complete crap, and that all reform advocates just wanted to get stoned and watch Cheech and Chong movies. I have had to radically rethink my worldview because of this.

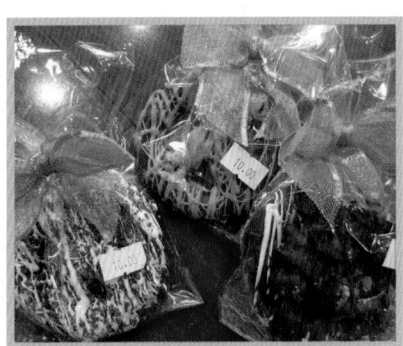

[MEDICATIONS] WOULD ACTUALLY EXACERBATE MY ISSUES OR TURN ME INTO A ZOMBIE.

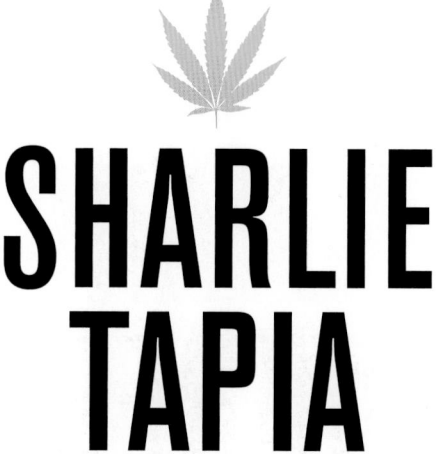

SHARLIE TAPIA

Age 21 / **Addiction, Depression, Anxiety** / Phoenix, Arizona

I'm a 21-year-old mother to the sweetest baby ever.

But when I was about 15, I fell into the pool of opiate addiction, starting with pills (Oxycontin) and ending with IV heroin. At 18, I found out I was pregnant. I had already planned on quitting, but the pregnancy made it official—I was done.

I've been clean for more than two years now, and cannabis helped me heal. On the days I really craved the hard stuff, cannabis helped me get it off my mind. I'd smoke and forget the feeling of want-ing to use. I use cannabis when I absolutely need it. I have a medical card because I have a son and I can't take any risks. It has saved me from addiction, depression, anxiety and ADHD. I don't even smoke it every day because some days I truly am happy that I don't need it.

Cannabis helps those who are in hiding because diseases such as addiction, anxiety, depression and ADHD are, for the most part, suffered in silence. We may look OK on the outside, but on the inside, it's a whole different story.

ON THE DAYS I REALLY CRAVED THE HARD STUFF, CANNABIS HELPED ME GET IT OFF MY MIND.

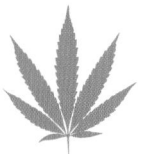

STAN RUTNER

Age 82 / **Stage 4 Lung Cancer, Metastatic Brain Tumor** / Santa Rosa, California

As told by his daughter, Corinne Malanca.

My story begins in 2011, the day after the Super Bowl. My father came over to have a chat with me. My heart sank when he told me that he was just diagnosed with stage-four lung cancer. He hadn't smoked since the 1980s. He had a good attitude—he told me it had been a great life and if he had a year or two, he was thankful. He entered right away into a program of six straight weeks of chemotherapy. It was tough, but he made it through. Ten days later, once he finished his chemo, he started to slur his words and we became worried he might have had a small stroke. It was at that point he was diagnosed with a brain tumor. It was a metastasis from the lungs and was located on the brain stem.

It was heart wrenching to see my parents have to go through this. Dad was now thrown into 10 straight days of full-brain radiation. Once he finished the radiation, he started declining rapidly and ended up in the hospital with a fever, which turned out to be radiation pneumonitis. Once he returned home he was bedridden and on full-time oxygen. I saw him wither away before my eyes. He could barely walk, only if to go to the bathroom. He was barely eating or drinking fluids. We had an appointment with the oncologist shortly thereafter. Dad wanted to know how much time he had. The doctor told us that when lung

176

NINE MONTHS AFTER STARTING THE CANNABIS TREATMENT, WE RECEIVED AN EMAIL FROM MY MOM. SHE WAS EXCITED TO SHARE MY DAD'S FIRST SCANS AFTER HIS GRIM PROGNOSIS OF WEEKS TO LIVE. THE REPORT READ, "NO EVIDENCE OF RECURRENT DISEASE."

cancer metastasizes to the brain, the prognosis is about six months, but, because of his setbacks with pneumonia, he had only weeks. We got my dad home and put him back to bed. Mom and I later talked and she said she was prepared for him to go any day.

In that meeting with the oncologist, we asked about legal medical marijuana. We had no experience with marijuana but had heard that it would increase his appetite and help with depression. The hospital doctor immediately wrote up a recommendation. I was deemed his caregiver and was immediately thrown into a

world that I had no idea how to navigate. We chose a coconut oil- and cannabis-infused capsule, so that we could freeze it and cut it. My mind was put as ease as we began to give my dad a half of a capsule every morning. At this point, my family was focusing on his quality of life. Hospice was brought in since it looked as though my dad was weeks, if not days, away from the end of his life. However, as soon as we started the marijuana capsules, my dad began to eat like a teenage boy. The results were almost immediate. His strength started to return, he was more talkative, and he

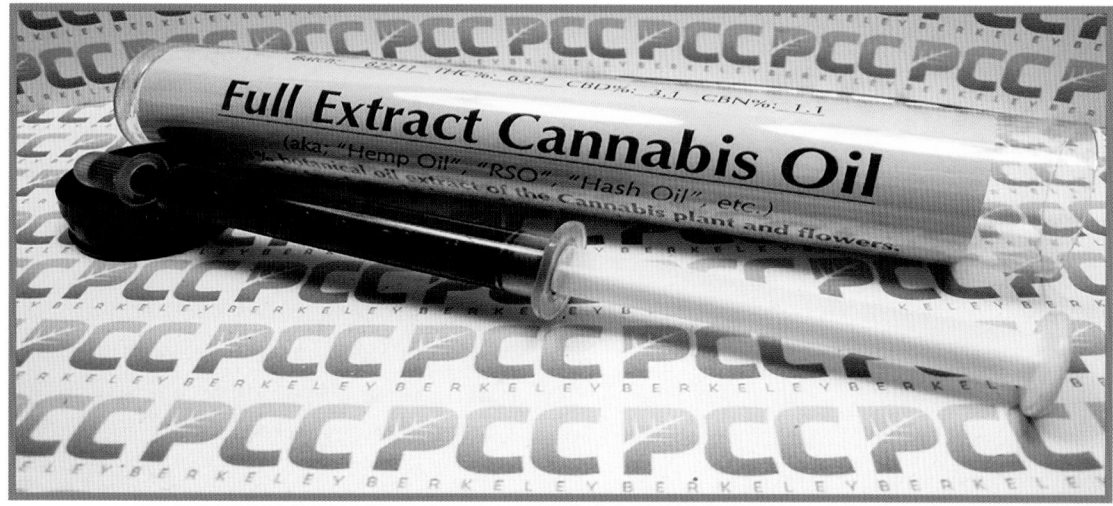

loved food again. Dad was back on his computer managing his properties and connecting with friends. He had more energy and was barely using any oxygen any longer—sometimes he went all day without it. After 10 days, the oxygen machine was in the closet for good.

My husband and I realized the need for medical cannabis information and education while offering support to families like ours. In turn, we founded United Patients Group. Since my dad is a retired dentist, he read every report, study or article on cannabis killing cancer.

After six months on the cannabis/coconut oil capsule, my dad said, "Maybe I have a chance, maybe I should try this oil everyone is talking about." In turn, we added a tiny dose of FECO (full-extract cannabis oil) under the tongue one hour before bed, a minute dose compared to the industry suggestions. This is all we ever gave him—half a capsule around 10 a.m. and a drop of FECO oil (the size of the ball on the head of a pin) before bed.

Nine months after starting the cannabis treatment, we received an email from my mom. She was excited to share my dad's first scans after his grim prognosis of weeks to live. The report read, "NO EVIDENCE OF RECURRENT DISEASE." We would never have believed it unless we saw it ourselves. Dad has had about five scans since then and it is now about four-plus years later and he is still cancer free. His oncologist still calls him the "Miracle Man" but we know it was no miracle.

Today my father has done a lot traveling, strength and balance classes, horseback riding, and walking. He enjoys a full life at 82 years young. Most importantly he made it to Montana to walk me down the aisle. Dad never thought that he would make it to that day, but lo and behold, he continued on the cannabis oil and is still in remission. Sept. 21, 2013, will go down in our history book. I knew that as soon as those barn doors opened and our wedding guests saw my father and me standing there, we would all fall apart.

My parents live at a senior community in Northern California and pride themselves on educating the other "inmates," as my parents call them, who live at their residence. My husband John and I were well received as we conducted a lecture on the benefits of cannabis and the process to get relief. It was a packed house and, in turn, many have gotten their cannabis cards. They are thrilled at the relief they have experienced and how they can function normally.

Dad now enjoys giving interviews and photo shoots—he has done many. The one that got him the most notoriety was his article in *Culture Magazine*. Mom and dad are very proud to be a part of the education process. It is rewarding for them to see people they know feeling better and hearing the remission stories that have come their direction. It's a good life, and it is cancer free.

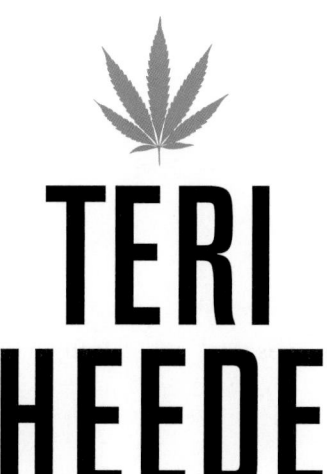

TERI HEEDE

Age 60 / **Multiple Sclerosis** / Makakilo, Hawai'i

Multiple Sclerosis is an immune system disorder, which means my body thinks there is something inside me that needs to be destroyed—only it happens to be the myelin sheath that surrounds the nerves.

Think of it like an electrical cord like the ones in your home, and imagine that the cover on the electrical cord just starts to dissolve, leaving the copper inside exposed. That is MS. The destruction creates lesions in the brain and on the spinal column, and eventually the lesions on the brain become black holes. There is no cure, and my symptoms include—but are by no means limited to—vision problems, mobility issues, and incontinence.

There are enough pills and suppositories to fill a laundry basket. As a direct result of indigestion of pharmaceuticals,

I developed something called "watermelon stomach." That means when they take a camera and look into my stomach, the walls have strange striations that resemble a watermelon because the pills ate the lining away and my stomach is permanently damaged. The damage extends up my esophagus, and they have removed pre-cancerous cells, so now I also have what is called Barrett's Esophagus Syndrome and have regular dates with my gastroenterologist.

A few years ago, in absolute desperation, injectable interferon was prescribed. Needles. When you have to deal with stuff like this, it is truly a "suck it up and act like an adult" moment. This was especially hard to suck up because there is no scientific evidence to support that taking interferon will delay or

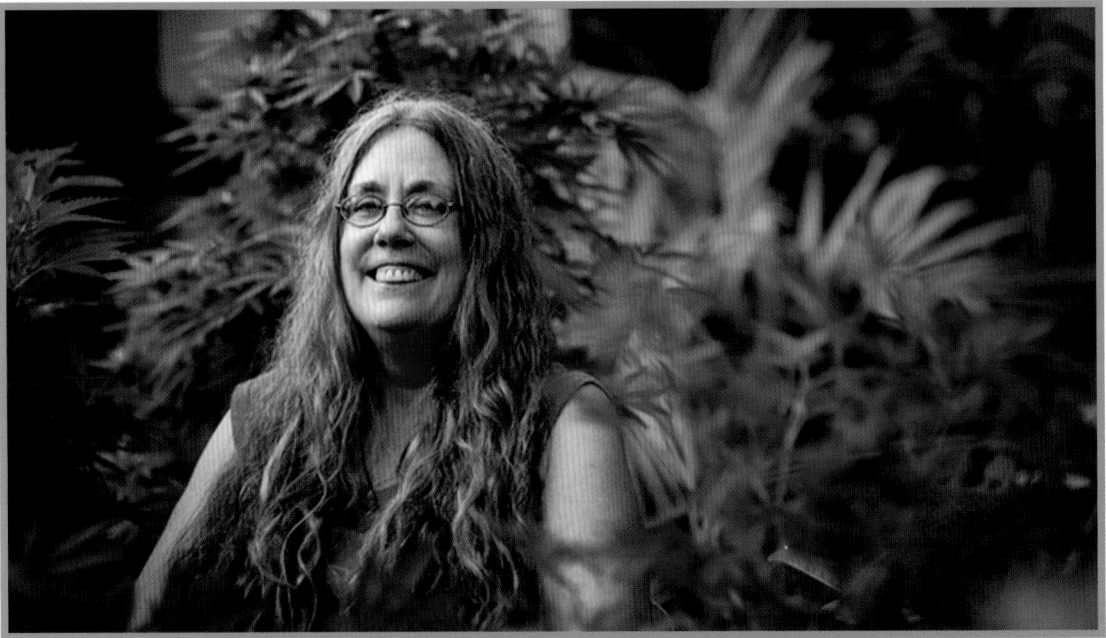

I LOOKED HIM RIGHT IN THE EYE AND SAID, "LET'S TALK ABOUT MARIJUANA." ... I WAS WALKING AGAIN WITHOUT ANY DEVICES WITHIN SIX MONTHS.

improve the symptoms of MS, but they think it might help. It took them three times a week subcutaneously until the side effects from the shots became so severe that I changed to a once-a-week intramuscular injection. Bigger needles. My side effects became even more severe (reactions at the injection site, rigors, fatigue and flu-like symptoms) and more deadly. My liver has now been damaged by the interferon. Remember that I have an autoimmune disorder, so this is not a good thing.

I remember the first time I discussed the use of cannabis with a doctor. I had

not been able to walk for a year. This doctor had served for a time as a doctor in a hospital that specialized in MS patients. My symptoms were progressively worsening, and I literally had fallen down and was not getting back up. Sitting with my grocery bag full of pills and watching him fill out another prescription, I looked him right in the eye and said, "Let's talk about marijuana." He folded his hands on top of my medical record and said, "Let's talk." I was walking again without any devices within six months.

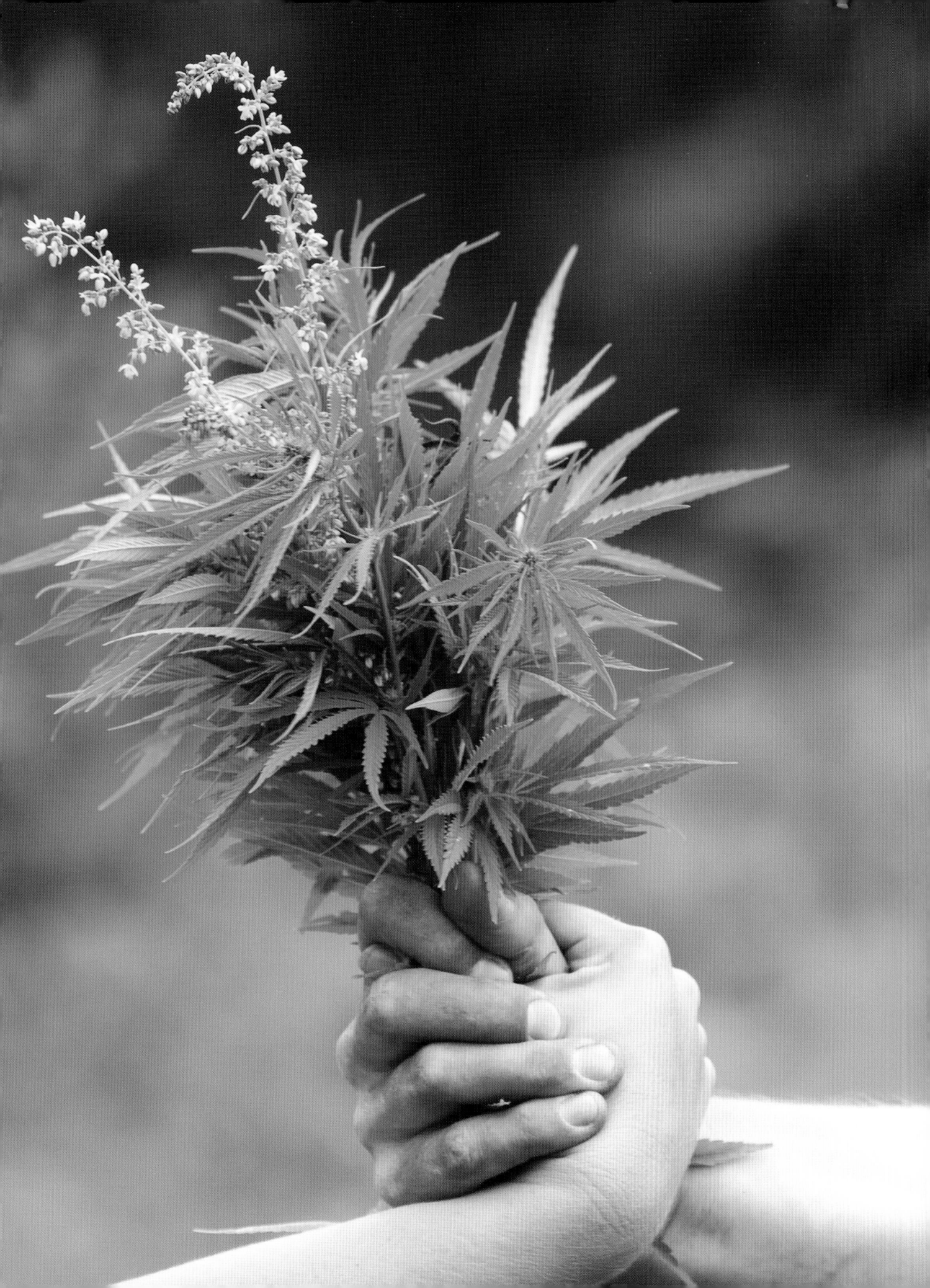

ACKNOWLEDGEMENTS

This book owes a great deal to the people who supported it along the way.

I extend my sincerest thanks and appreciation to Aaron Kase, whose hard work and journalistic talents are behind all of the book's sidebars; April Short, the brilliant writer/editor who is responsible for my writing of this book; Christa Martin, for her skill, smarts and incredible generosity; everyone at Reset.me for their encouragement and assistance; Carol and Kevin Limbach, who never hesitate to help; and Josh Becker, whose endless support made it all possible.

Most of all, I'd like to thank the brave individuals who shared their deeply personal stories with me, and trusted me, in turn, to share them with you. This book is truly theirs.

FOR MORE INFORMATION

- Illegally Healed: illegallyhealed.com

- NORML: norml.org

- Americans for Safe Access: safeaccessnow.org

- Realm of Caring: theroc.us

- Drug Police Alliance: DrugPolicy.org

- Reset.me: Reset.me

- Marijuana Policy Project: mpp.org

- Veterans for Medical Cannabis: veteransformedicalmarijuana.org

- Cannabis as Medicine: medicalcannabis.com

- Cannabis Medical Dictionary: cannabismedicaldictionary.com

- American Alliance for Medical Cannabis: letfreedomgrow.com

- Cannabis Consumers Campaign: cannabisconsumers.org

- Medical Marijuana ProCon: medicalmarijuana.procon.org

- United Patients Group: unitedpatientsgroup.com

- Multidisciplinary Association for Psychedelic Studies (MAPS): maps.org/research-archive/mmj

About the Author

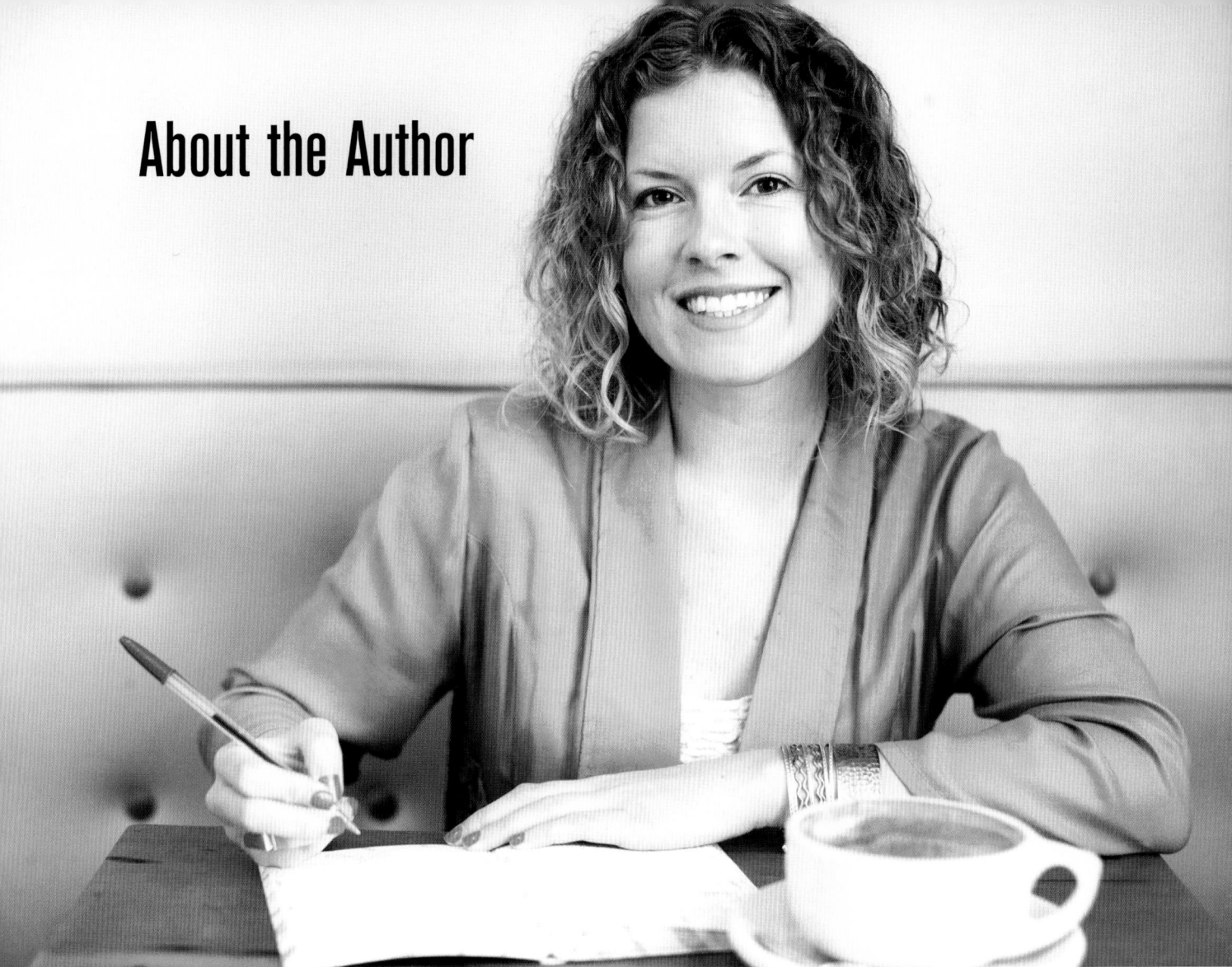

Elizabeth Limbach is an award-winning journalist, former weekly newspaper editor, and current magazine editor living in Santa Cruz, California.

Her work has been published by TheAtlantic.com, Ms. Magazine, Parade, Sierra Magazine, American Way, Alternet.org, and E – The Environmental Magazine, among others.

Find her online at elizabethlimbach.com.

APPENDIX

ALS: Amyotrophic lateral sclerosis, better known as ALS or Lou Gehrig's disease, is a neurodegenerative disease characterized by a hardening in the spinal cord that prevents messages from the brain from reaching the body. Cannabis can help protect the nerves that control body movement by stimulating the endocannabinoid system, as well as relieve symptoms of ALS. Studies have shown cannabis can delay motor impairment and prolong survival in animals, but non-anecdotal research on humans has been stymied by federal regulations. Sources: ALS Association, Americans for Safe Access.

ANXIETY & DEPRESSION: Anxiety and depression are mental disorders associated with crippling despondency or worry that makes it difficult for sufferers to interact with other people or enjoy life. Studies have shown that marijuana users have less depressed mood indicators than non-smokers, and suicide rates are lower in states that allow medical cannabis. Cannabinoid receptors have also been found in the area of the brain that regulates anxiety in mice, providing evidence to back up anecdotal reports of people who say that marijuana helps them reduce their anxiety. Sources: Medical Marijuana ProCon, Medical Daily.

CANCER & CANNABIS: Cancer is caused when abnormal cells in the human body multiply uncontrollably, resulting in tumors that can rapidly spread to other parts of the body and ultimately kill the patient. Medical marijuana has long been used to reduce nausea and promote appetite in people undergoing cancer treatment, but recent research shows that cannabis can also be useful for treating the cancer itself. A study published in 2014 showed that THC can cause cancer cells in mice to self-destruct, and can slow down the advance of brain and breast cancer. Other preliminary research and anecdotal reports suggest that cannabis is also useful against colorectal cancer, skin cancer and prostate cancer. Researchers suspect that marijuana exhibits these cancer-fighting properties because it stimulates the body's endocannabinoid system, which, among other functions, controls the recycling of cell materials, an essential component of anti-tumor responses. Sources: American Cancer Society, Leafscience.com, NORML.

CBD: CBD is short for cannabidiol, one of the primary active compounds in cannabis. CBD is thought to be responsible for many of the medical benefits of cannabis, and has shown efficacy against arthritis, multiple sclerosis (MS), epilepsy, inflammation, anxiety and many other ailments. The compound has also shown promise in fighting cancer. Oils derived from CBD-rich marijuana strains lack the psychoactive component that the plant is known for, and are therefore popular for treating illness in children and for people who don't like feeling high or stoned. Sources: ProjectCBD.org, leafscience.com.

CHARLOTTE'S WEB: Charlotte's Web is a form of non-psychoactive cannabis oil used to treat seizures in children. The oil was named after Charlotte Figi, a 5-year-old girl who suffered from uncontrollable epileptic seizures. The only treatment that worked was a certain strain of CBD oil, which her mother said stopped 99.9 percent of the seizures. After Charlotte's story was featured in the 2013 CNN documentary *Weed*, other families started seeking the treatment, and Charlotte's Web is now sold commercially to help other epileptic children. The oil is also the inspiration behind the Charlotte's Web Medical Access Act, a bill under consideration by Congress that would remove the federal prohibition on marijuana strains that have little or no THC and therefore don't cause users to feel high. Source: Realm of Caring Foundation, Reset.me, Epilepsy Foundation of Colorado.

COMPARING SIDE EFFECTS: Like any medicine, cannabis has side effects in addition to the treatment of a specific illness. Most notably, smoking or ingesting cannabis with moderate-to-high THC levels causes a user to feel high, or stoned, which can result in euphoric feelings and can affect short-term memory, concentration, sensory perception and coordination. Marijuana may also cause paranoia, anxiety and fear in some users, but cannot cause death by overdose. By comparison, pharmaceutical drugs commonly prescribed for depression and other mental disorders have a raft of potential side effects. For example:

•**KLONOPIN** (Clonazepam) is a benzodiazepine with numerous common side effects, including weakness, headaches, body pain, breathing trouble, depression, sleep disturbances, diarrhea, constipation, and blurred vision. Klonopin users can also experience confusion and hallucinations, and exhibit unusual risk-taking behavior. The drug has serious habit-forming potential and can lead to suicidal thoughts. Overdoses can be fatal.

• **SEROQUEL** (Quetiapine) is a psychotropic medication with its own array of side effects. People who take Seroquel sometimes deal with mood or behavior changes, chills, cold sweats, confusion, upset stomach, nausea, vomiting, dizziness, drowsiness and more. For older people with dementia, it can provoke heart failure and stroke. It can also create fetal health problems for pregnant women and can pass through breast milk into a nursing baby. Young people who take Seroquel sometimes have suicidal thoughts, and overdoses are potentially fatal.

• **ZOLOFT** (Sertraline) is a selective serotonin reuptake inhibitor commonly prescribed for depression. Among other side effects are sleepiness, nervousness, insomnia, dizziness, nausea, headache, diarrhea, constipation and stomach pain. Some people experience aggressive reactions, paranoia, hallucination and psychotic disorders, and it can also cause various forms of sexual dysfunction. Zoloft has been known to provoke suicidal thoughts in users, particularly teenagers. Overdoses can be fatal. Sources: Rxlist.com, NORML, Live Science, Drugs.com.

COMPASSIONATE USE: Compassionate use is when a drug or treatment that has not been approved by the U.S. Food and Drug Administration is used with permission, outside of official clinical trials. A small handful of patients were permitted to use, and were supplied with, cannabis by the federal government starting in the 1970s after patient Robert Randall successfully argued in court that he needed marijuana to control his glaucoma. The compassionate investigational new drug program for marijuana was closed to new patients in 1992, and today only four people still receive cannabis from the government. Source: U.S. Food and Drug Administration, medicalcannabis.com.

ENDOCANNABINOID SYSTEM: The human body is built to respond to cannabis through what is called the endocannabinoid system, comprised of cannabinoid receptors in the brain and throughout the body. Humans and other animals naturally produce substances to stimulate the cannabinoid receptors, which are essential to maintaining the body's internal systems and helping us respond to ever changing and sometimes dangerous outside stimuli. The endocannabinoid system regulates numerous functions, such as inflammatory responses and the recycling of cell materials, and is important for controlling pain, promoting healing and marshaling anti-tumor responses. Numerous compounds in marijuana, such as THC and CBD, also stimulate our cannabinoid receptors, which is thought to be why cannabis has so many medicinal applications. Scientists are still working to broaden our understanding of how the endocannabinoid system works, but it's become clear that it is essential to maintaining good health. Source: NORML.

EPILEPSY: Epilepsy is a neurological disorder most commonly associated with seizures. Extreme cases can provoke hundreds of uncontrollable seizures per day. Studies and anecdotal evidence suggest that cannabis, and CBD oil in particular,

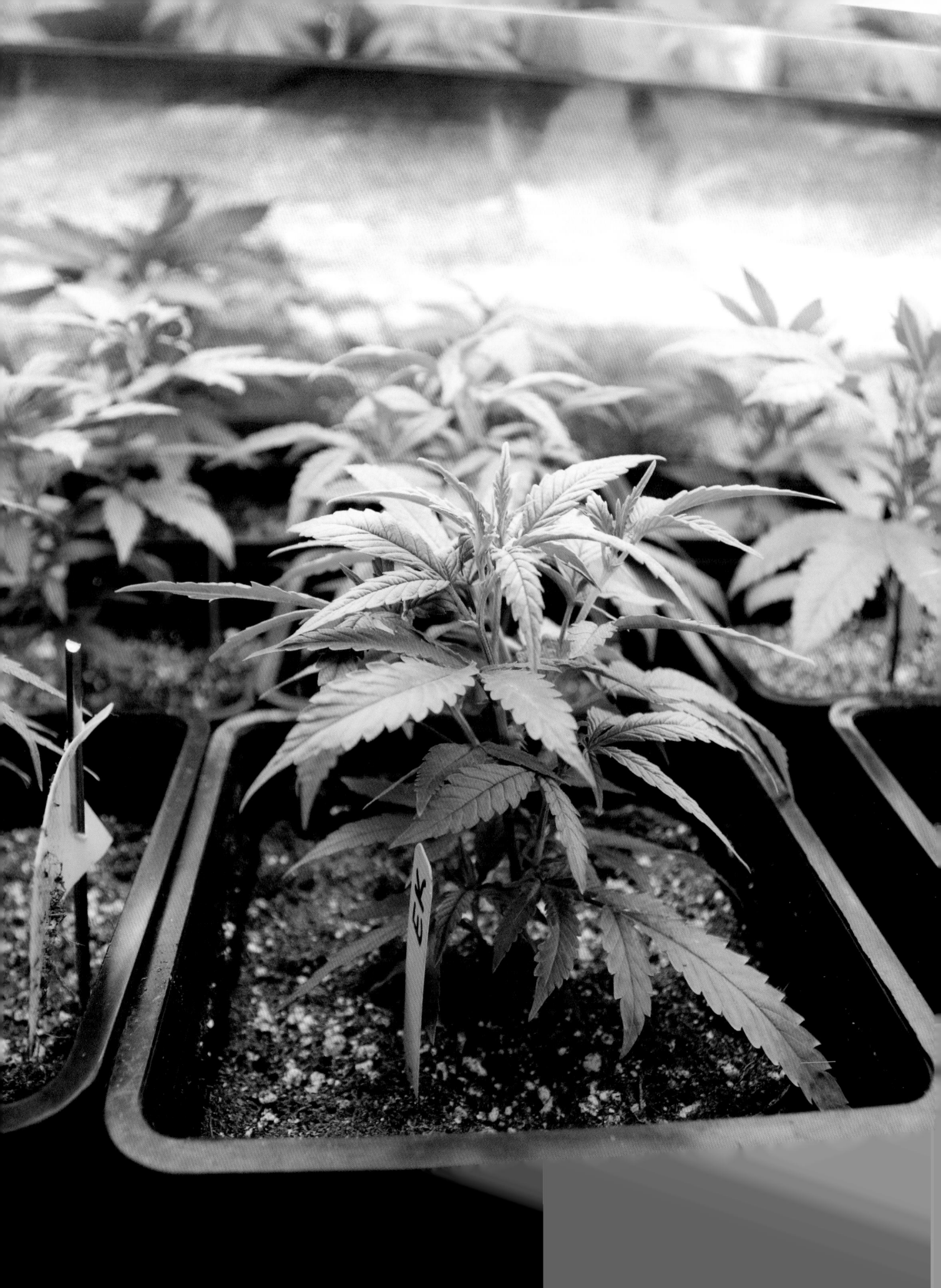

can help control seizures in some cases where pharmaceutical interventions have failed to make an impact. The treatment has shown great promise in helping epileptic children live normal lives. Sources: Epilepsy Foundation of Colorado, Realm of Caring Foundation.

FIBROMYALGIA: Fibromyalgia is a disease that causes fatigue and musculoskeletal pain, particularly in the neck, spine, shoulders and hips. There is no known cure, but many patients find marijuana helps relieve pain and other symptoms. A 2014 online survey sponsored by the National Pain Foundation found that patients said medical marijuana was better at treating fibromyalgia symptoms than FDA-approved drugs, with 62 percent of respondents saying it was "very effective." Sources: National Pain Report, NORML.

LEGALIZATION: About 53 percent of Americans believe that marijuana should be legal, according to a Pew poll released in April 2015. The same poll found that about half of all Americans have tried marijuana. A Harris Poll released in May 2015 reported that 81 percent of adults in the United States are in favor of legalizing marijuana for medical use. A survey conducted by WebMD in 2014 found that 67 percent of doctors believe that marijuana should be a medical option for patients.

MEDICAL NECESSITY: In states where medical marijuana is not legal, patients who are prosecuted for possessing or consuming cannabis may argue in court that their use of the substance is medically necessary. A defendant making this claim would acknowledge that he or she broke the law, but argue that cannabis use was the "lesser evil" compared to succumbing to a debilitating illness. Medical necessity arguments need to show that there is no legal alternative treatment for the medical condition in question, and require testimony from a medical expert. Source: NORML.org.

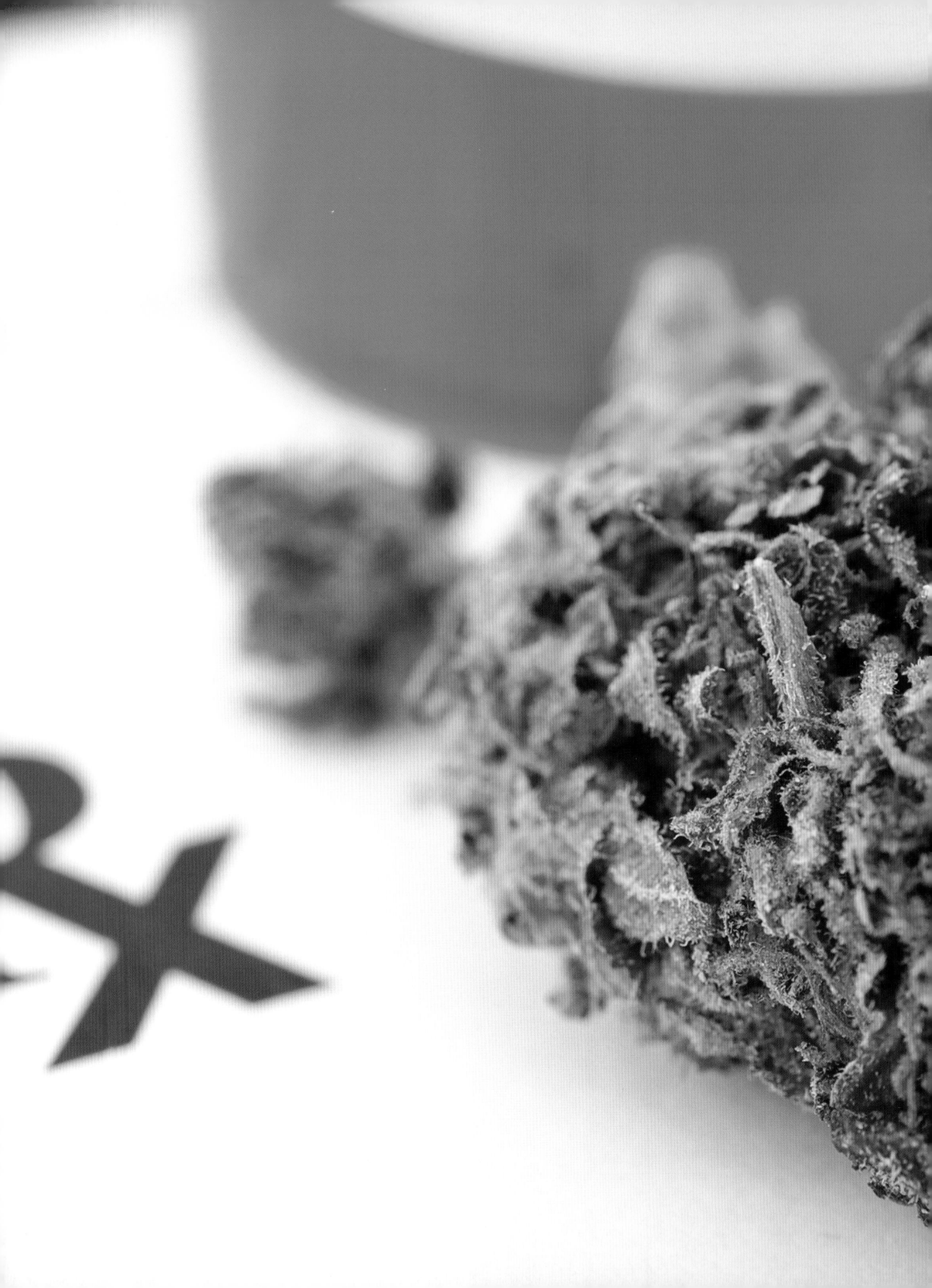

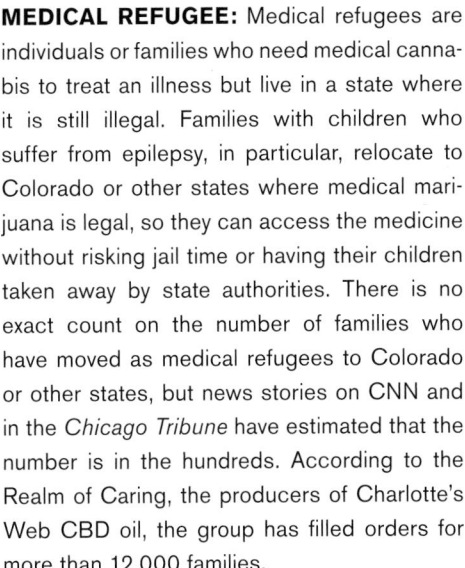

MEDICAL REFUGEE: Medical refugees are individuals or families who need medical cannabis to treat an illness but live in a state where it is still illegal. Families with children who suffer from epilepsy, in particular, relocate to Colorado or other states where medical marijuana is legal, so they can access the medicine without risking jail time or having their children taken away by state authorities. There is no exact count on the number of families who have moved as medical refugees to Colorado or other states, but news stories on CNN and in the *Chicago Tribune* have estimated that the number is in the hundreds. According to the Realm of Caring, the producers of Charlotte's Web CBD oil, the group has filled orders for more than 12,000 families.

MS: Multiple sclerosis, or MS, is a disease that occurs when the immune system reacts against the central nervous system, damaging the brain's ability to send and receive information to and from the body. Extensive scientific evidence shows that cannabis can help control pain and other symptoms associated with MS, and some studies suggest that the plant can limit the progression of the disease. Sources: National Multiple Sclerosis Society, NORML.

PATENTS: There are about 1,660 patents in the United States related to cannabis, according to Google Patent Search. The U.S. Department of Health and Human Services was granted a patent in 2003 for "Cannabinoids as antioxidants and neuroprotectants," which acknowledges their utility against stroke, Alzheimer's disease, Parkinson's disease and dementia, according to the U.S. Patent and Trademark Office.

PROHIBITION: At the dawn of the 20th century, cannabis was used widely in medicinal products in the United States. However, prejudice against Mexican immigrants who used marijuana recreationally led to a backlash against the plant by the 1930s, and numerous states instituted prohibition policies. The anti-marijuana propaganda film *Reefer Madness*, released in 1936, reinforced the false premise that smoking marijuana provoked crime and other deviant behavior. The Marijuana Tax Act of 1937 acted as a de-facto federal ban, which was reinforced by stricter sentencing laws in subsequent decades, and the Controlled Substances Act, enacted in 1970, placed cannabis in Schedule I, the most restrictive category. In recent decades, however, the tide has shifted, after California became the first state to legalize medical marijuana in 1996. Currently, 23 states plus Washington, D.C., allow medical usage of cannabis, and four states have legalized it outright. Sources: PBS, Drug Policy Alliance.

PTSD: Post-traumatic stress disorder occurs when people who have experienced trauma find themselves reliving uncontrollable fear, helplessness and distress when they are reminded of the incident. The disorder frequently occurs in war veterans but can affect anyone who has experienced or witnessed assault or trauma. Cannabis can help control anxiety and depression in PTSD patients, and emerging research even suggests that it can deactivate traumatic memories by stimulating the endocannabinoid system. Sources: Veterans for Medical Marijuana, Leafly.com.

RICK SIMPSON OIL: In 2003, Rick Simpson discovered that hemp oil was an effective cure for his basil cell carcinoma skin cancer. Since then he has spread the word to encourage others to benefit from the medicine as he has. Simpson starred in the documentary *Run From the Cure*, and provides free instructions on how to create the oil on his website PhoenixTears.ca. Simpson considers his oil a preventative medicine that promotes full-body healing, and can help ward off diseases like diabetes, cancer and multiple sclerosis (MS) before they start. Source: PhoenixTears.ca.

SCHEDULE I: The federal Controlled Substance Act defines Schedule I substances as "drugs with no currently accepted medical use and a high potential for abuse." This listing means that the substances in question are strictly forbidden by federal law, and research on them requires special, difficult-to-acquire permission to perform. Cannabis is categorized as a Schedule I substance despite overwhelming evidence of its numerous medical benefits and no evidence that it is harmful or toxic. As a result, between 1999 and 2014, the federal government approved only 16 independent studies of medical marijuana on humans, according to *Time* magazine.

STATE LAWS: Twenty-three states plus Washington, D.C., currently have medical marijuana laws, according to the National Conference of State Legislatures. An additional 15 states allow limited use of CBD oil for medicinal use or as a legal defense. So far, Colorado, Washington, Oregon, Alaska and Washington, D.C., have legalized marijuana for recreational use, according to NORML. As of this writing, Pennsylvania has a measure to legalize medical marijuana pending a vote, while 17 other states introduced but failed to pass medical marijuana laws in 2015, according to ProCon.org. The United States Congress is also considering one piece of legislation that would remove low-THC concentrations of cannabis from the federal definition of marijuana, and another that would move marijuana off Schedule I of the Controlled Substances Act entirely.

SYNTHETIC CANNABIS: There is a legal pharmaceutical synthetic cannabis product on the market called Marinol, or Dronabinol, which doctors can prescribe to AIDS and cancer patients to stimulate the appetite and control nausea. Marinol contains synthetic THC and is approved by the U.S. Food and Drug Administration. However, many practitioners still recommend natural cannabis products because synthetics such as Marinol are missing many of the other beneficial compounds, like CBD, that are found in marijuana. Not only do compounds like CBD have their own medicinal value, but they are also thought to act synergistically with THC to produce even more benefits, which are lost when the THC is produced in a lab in the absence of the other compounds. Source: NORML, U.S. National Library of Medicine.

THC: Tetrahydrocannabinol, or THC, is the main active component in cannabis and the source of the high, or stoned, feeling in users. The compound is created when cannabis buds and other plant bits are heated, which is one reason smoking and vaporizing marijuana are popular ways to consume the plant. THC binds to cannabinoid receptors in the brain and can affect memory, pleasure, concentration and other functions. The compound has proven useful to combat nausea and pain, and to stimulate the appetite of people suffering from serious illnesses like cancer. Other studies suggest it can also help treat amyotrophic lateral sclerosis (ALS), multiple sclerosis (MS), Alzheimer's, Crohn's disease, cancer and more. Sources: LiveScience.com, UnitedPatientsGroup.com.

THCA: Tetrahydrocannabinolic acid is a precursor to THC that is found in live cannabis plants before they are subjected to heat. THCA is not psychoactive, and is collected from freshly harvested plants before they start to dry. Juicing raw cannabis plants, for example, is a popular way to obtain the compound. Preliminary research suggests THCA has numerous benefits, including anti-inflammatory, neuroprotective, anti-nausea, anti-seizure and anti-cancer properties. Sources: Leafly.com, UnitedPatientsGroup.com.

THCV: THCV is short for tetrahydrocannabivarin, another beneficial compound found in cannabis plants. Many cannabis strains have only trace amounts of THCV. The compound is psychoactive and affects the same brain receptors as THC, but the buzz it creates is considered to be more clear-headed and euphoric.

Initial research suggests that THCV can be useful as an appetite suppressant, and also for stimulating bone growth, preventing panic attacks, and helping mitigate the effects of diabetes and Alzheimer's. Source: Leafly.com.

TINCTURE: Cannabis tinctures are made by soaking dried cannabis in alcohol, which extracts the THC and creates a liquid that preserves the psychoactive and medicinal properties of the original plant. Tinctures are taken orally or placed under the tongue and take effect relatively quickly. They are popular among patients who don't like to smoke or cannot smoke cannabis.

VAPORIZER: Vaporizers use heat to turn cannabis buds or other plant materials into a vapor that can be inhaled, as opposed to applying fire to the plant to create smoke. Many people prefer to use vaporizers because they don't create harmful toxins that accompany smoke, and therefore are suspected to be safer for your lungs. Vaporizing creates a near-instantaneous effect, similar to smoking, and it preserves more THC and other beneficial compounds than smoking does, so users need less marijuana to achieve the same results.

VETERANS & CANNABIS: Soldiers returning from Iraq, Afghanistan and other combat zones often suffer from ailments that cannabis can help treat, like pain, anxiety and post-traumatic stress disorder. However, doctors who work in the Veterans Administration system are barred by federal law from recommending marijuana to their patients. As a result, veterans who rely on the VA system for their healthcare have no way to legally access a medicine that can help them control their symptoms. Some veterans groups are advocating to change the rule, and Congress is currently considering a bill that would allow VA doctors to recommend medical marijuana to patients in states where it is legal. Sources: Veterans for Medical Cannabis Access, Drug Policy Alliance.

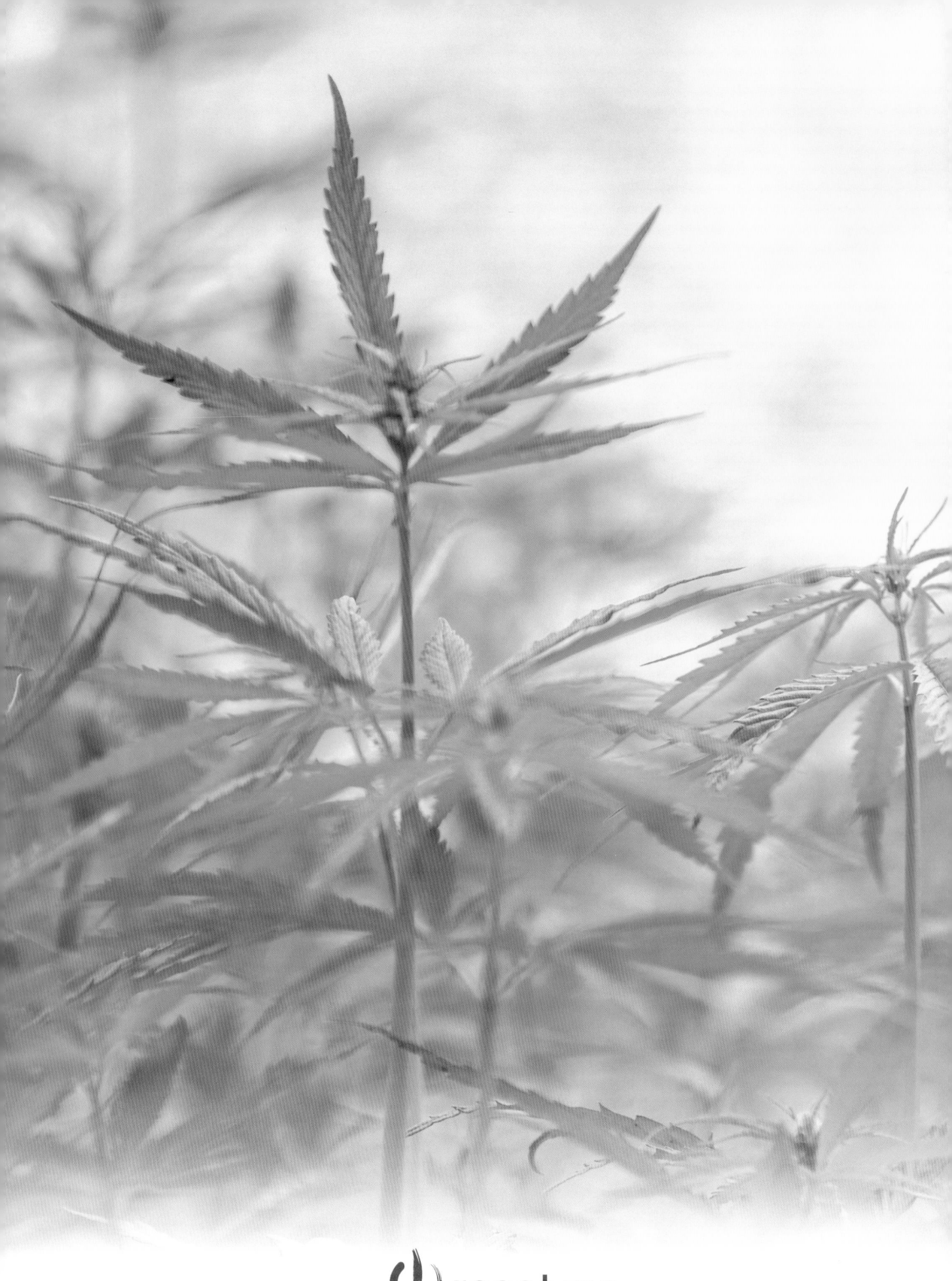

reset.me